Hiding in Plain Sight

The Truth About Trauma, Service, and the Way Forward

Doug White

Copyright © 2024 by Doug White. *Tell This Story*.

All rights reserved. No part of this publication may be reproduced, distributed, or transmitted in any form or by any means, without prior written permission.

Printed in the United States of America

First Edition

ISBN (print): 979-8-3304-3328-5

ISBN (ebook): 979-8-3304-4379-6

For information on bulk orders or to contact the author, visit www.DougWhiteOfficial.com.

Dedication

It is my opinion, and I am certainly not alone in this view, that the loved ones of first responders and service members are brave and bold. They have bound themselves to us and, by extension, are bound to our service. We leave them for our eight- to twenty-four-hour shifts and months-long deployments, and they are left wondering if we are coming home. Now, I know, like the first responder, that this is not a forethought of every waking moment, but it is a reality and is visited in the minds of our loved ones as we place ourselves in harm's way.

As partners, they hold us together and have a front-row seat as we walk toward the edge and stare into the abyss. They hold on dearly to the person they once knew, hoping for them to return. Our children are the recipients of secondary or vicarious trauma and the remains of the day we carry with us. Quick to anger, quick to speak, and quick to disengage, our actions take a toll. For these reasons, the following pages are dedicated to them.

First, to my wife Michelle, my hero, shield, and retreat, who, despite my best efforts to live in the shadows and conceal every fracture in my soul, always saw the light shining through the cracks. She loved me fiercely, even when I made it difficult. To my children, who are now in their late teens and will learn more about their father should they decide to read the following pages. While I love them more than my next breath, they bore the brunt of my trauma and decisions undeservingly. Something I can never take back, but I hope to provide the understanding, and I may receive their grace in time.

To the responders, dispatchers, veterans, and those actively serving in the armed forces, all trauma and all issues are based on perspective. This doesn't mean you're not hard or unaware; it just means there's a limit. Each of you has a front-row seat and often plays an active role in human tragedy. You may be present during the worst moments of someone's life and then again and again. When the job is done, or the mission is over, you are left with the story. These can be haunting snapshots through time, a vivid and frightening collage chronicling a life of service.

Disclaimer

The following pages are narrated from my vantage point—my perspective, feelings, and experiences. While I have ensured their completeness, the vignettes within should not be relied upon as material or circumstantial evidence of a crime or civil action. They are subject to the limitations of memory, with gaps filled in by decades of compounding traumatic experiences. The vignettes and cases in the following pages were concluded through further investigation by others following my involvement.

My recollection of these events may be difficult to read and could trigger memories of events experienced by the reader. These events are gritty, visceral, and gut-wrenching, much like my reactions. I do not recount them to establish an acceptable baseline for trauma or to compare my experience with anyone else's; they are intended to paint a picture for the reader and my recognition of opportunities missed. What's more, they were part of the process of my writing this book.

I am not a clinician. This collection of stories, the hard

lessons learned, and the way I found forward are not meant to, and will not, provide diagnoses. It is not a substitute for professional help and guidance as you navigate your path. I hope the reader discovers something relatable that pulls them from the shadows and sets them on the path to healing.

Contents

Foreword Adam Davis	ix
Preface Michelle White	xiii
Introduction	xv
1. When it All Began	1
2. Off We Go, Into the Wild Blue Yonder	8
3. A Rebuilding Season	13
4. The Office	18
5. September 11, 2001	23
6. Back at the Office	31
7. Uncle Jimmy, the Bear, and the Devil	37
8. Scene 1, Death From Below	42
9. Scene 2, I Couldn't Save Them August-September 1998	46
10. Scene 3, Date Day and the Wandering Eye	49
11. Scene 4, The Airmen and New Boots-1999	52
12. Scene 5, The Dead Cat and Moral Injury	57
13. Scene 6, Keep Your Finger Off the Trigger	61
14. Scene 7, We Went to Work	64
15. Scene 8, The Weekend: The Devil, the Duffel, and the Angel	76
16. Scene 9, I Never Knew Her Name	87
17. Scene 10, The Sound and The Screaming Eagle	90
18. Scene 11, A Simple Marker and Indelible Mark.	94
19. Leadership Opportunities	99
20. My Drive and the Cost	105
21. The Beginning of the End	118

22. The Days and Months After	141
23. Transitioning	156
24. What Can Be Done?	165
25. Growth	169
About Doug White	179
Notes	181

Foreword
Adam Davis

As I read *Hiding in Plain Sight*, I felt moments of anger and sadness, and there were many moments when I could relate to Doug's stories.

I believe that if you are a law enforcement officer or other first responder, you will experience the same thing.

Here's the reality: don't run from how you feel. Sit with it. Feel it. Then, attack that junk so you can heal.

I know this from my own experiences.

Since 2015, I have traveled across the United States, sharing the *Live Unconquered* message and my story of overcoming childhood trauma and suicidal ideations. I learned early on in the journey how many people there were who dealt with some of the things I battled, and there were many. When my latest book, *Unconquered*, was released in 2023, they came out of the shadows.

Many of us live just like that, cloaked in past pain, trauma, or some other challenge we are facing, living in the shadows of life instead of living life to the fullest. Trauma, pain, loss, grief,

Foreword

it all affects us differently, and we have been conditioned to "suck it up" or "push that stuff down" and move on.

I lived like that for a long time.

Living in the shadows becomes comfortable because, even with our pain, it's at least something we're familiar with in life.

So, we blend in with the crowd. We put on the facade, laugh, smile, and carry on with our daily duties so we don't disturb anyone else. We don't want to be a burden because we know others are also struggling with their own issues.

But what you're about to read will challenge you to step out of the shadows of pain and comfort and step into a journey of healing and abundant life.

However, I want to issue a word of caution to you as you proceed.

Do not take this flippantly. This is a field guide for healing. If you are in the beginning phases of your journey, learn from Doug's experiences. You don't have to wait until the end of your career to begin healing or live well.

You can begin now.

You can step out of the shadows today and into the light of a new way of life.

Carrying the trauma, the pain, and the deep wounds is not a badge of honor, and it's not a feather in our hats or another stripe on our sleeves. It's a demon that must be dealt with before it destroys every part of our lives.

Doug was, and is, a phenomenal leader. He is a man I'd follow into any situation, and I am grateful our paths have crossed. I am honored to write the foreword for this timely book, and one I hope *you* will take time to read, study, and apply.

We're all connected by pain. Why not start a new

connection today? One based on healing, wellness, and the strength we find in a new way of living?

Fight like hell for what matters most.

Live Unconquered!

Adam Davis
Bestselling Author, Speaker, Coach
www.TheAdamDavis.com

Preface
Michelle White

"The deepest love is the kind that can turn the darkest times into something beautiful."

— Unknown

Doug and I met just a few months before I turned 19. I quickly realized he was the man I wanted to build a future with. That realization scared the hell out of me, and I broke up with him. But Doug waited patiently, giving me the time I needed to find my way back to him. We were married two years later. Over the past 24 years of marriage, we've raised two incredible kids, celebrated career and personal successes, and shared countless adventures. We've faced challenges and navigated through difficult times, always united by our "us against the world" mentality. But when the struggle became "us against us," it took unfortunate events, prayer, and some therapy to help us find our way back.

I've been a law enforcement spouse for our entire marriage. When I said "I do," I knew it would mean years of shift work,

Preface

long hours, and dangerous situations. What I didn't realize was that it could also mean living with a spouse tormented by trauma, a man who became emotionally unavailable. This left me to take on the role of primary household administrator and default parent for most of our marriage. As a fiercely independent person, I took on those roles and owned them—but the resentment began to build as I watched Doug sink further and further away from me.

I watched the man I love struggle for years and did my best to support him. My years of therapy, sorting through my past trauma, gave me the tools to keep moving forward, but it was lonely and exhausting. Many nights, I found myself praying for his physical safety and praying even harder for him to heal from his invisible wounds.

This book is raw and vulnerable. I watched it unfold in real life and then witnessed Doug spend countless hours pouring his soul onto the page. I'm proud that this story is being told. I'm proud of my husband and his career. But most of all, I'm proud that we survived this journey together and have many beautiful years ahead.

To the struggling men and women reading this book: Don't shut out your loved ones. There is no safer place than the arms of someone who truly knows your heart and loves you. Don't struggle alone. Let them in—it's worth it.

To the men and women supporting someone who is struggling: Don't be afraid to speak up. I spent years wondering how to tell the man I love so deeply that he was broken. Divine intervention kept him alive, and I'm forever grateful that God was watching over him until I found the courage to ask him to seek counseling.

Introduction

What you will read in this book is far different from what I intended to write in the beginning. The initial content was a mixture of unsorted raw feelings, peppered with organized rants about my shortfalls and regrets, a blend of my perceived missed opportunities and comparing my journey to the journeys of others. Initially, my writing was fueled by undeserved imposter syndrome, shame, and chronic downplaying of the positive role I played in many lives during my more than thirty years of service to my country and community.

It was not until five months after I retired and put 77,000 words into this project that I realized the initial draft was the journal I should have kept for years but *never* took the time to do so. Honestly, I was not motivated because I thought journaling was pointless and would not serve me in any way. When it was suggested as a method of reflection or self-care, I dismissed it and laughed it off, claiming I was too lazy. Dismissive of the advice and self-deprecating in my response to

Introduction

any help offered, I eventually discovered that journaling was an effective way to get everything out. I was never honest with myself or my loved ones about my trauma, fears, the monster, or my insecurities hidden in the shadows, but I was very revealing to the blank slate presented by my laptop.

I sat down to *pen* the words to chronicle my experiences in service and found that the feelings poured from me. I could not type fast enough. I revealed feelings and thoughts never shared, much less examined meaningfully. I discovered experiences I previously dismissed as the cost of doing business or just another day at the office sparked a visceral churning in me that I had not felt since the moment they first occurred, and certainly nothing I experienced sitting in the safety of my home.

These feelings caused me to retreat and isolate myself as they had previously done. I stepped away from writing this book for weeks on end, not wanting to peel back the layers that would have ultimately allowed me to examine the events and see them in a way that would have allowed me to reframe them and possibly put them to rest.

I wasn't alone on this journey. My wife has accompanied me for 26 out of the 30 years of service and still does today. Two children were also present. Now in their late teens, they grew up in the shadow of my experiences and were exposed to trauma vicariously through me.

I read books published by other veterans and responders in the dead space created by not writing or journaling. I was trying to gain perspective or even the proper words to convey many of my thoughts. I found value in these stories; I found different ways to convey a message. I learned I was not alone; though our experiences may have been different, our physiological and psychological reactions to our experiences were similar.

This journey has taught me that time and distance offer perspective, a white space, free of chaos, in which to heal. In that space, I realized the importance of supporting, being vulnerable, and being accountable. In this space, I read my *journal*, what was to be a chronicle, my odyssey, and discovered that I had written myself as a victim or bystander in my *hero's journey*. I imagine this perspective directly resulted from straying from my purpose, allowing others to assign value to me and my career, leaving me vulnerable and somehow weaker.

Burning out, I waited for a profession and an organization to love me back, and when it did not, I was crushed. I was weakened due to a perceived organizational injustice or betrayal, leading me to give away my power and joy; this was where I built my house, and this is where I lived until I was pulled back from the edge.

Thoughts and Concepts: The Shadow, the Monster, Ego, and Persona

This section introduces key concepts that serve as a foundation for understanding my journey. The interpretation of the following concepts is based on my own perspective and understanding of the subject matter.

In the 20th century, Swiss psychiatrist and psychoanalyst Dr. Carl Jung proposed the idea of a collective unconscious, suggesting that this shared reservoir of the unconscious mind links every human.[1] This concept encompasses universal structures, patterns, symbols, and reactions common to people worldwide. Exploring some of Dr. Jung's core concepts is necessary to provide a framework for the terms I use in the following pages.

Dr. Carl Jung introduced the concept of the collective unconscious, a shared mental repository containing universal archetypes or templates for everyday human experiences and characters. These archetypes include heroes, villains, wise figures, and mothers, which exist in every individual's mind.[2] Jung's exploration of archetypes also underscores their relevance across cultures, linking individuals through shared unconscious symbols.

Jung also discussed the ego, which represents your conscious self and is responsible for thinking and decision-making. The persona functions as your outward mask, shaping the image you present in different social settings, such as work or with friends. Meanwhile, the shadow symbolizes your personality's hidden, darker aspects, where thoughts and emotions you may prefer to avoid, like fear, guilt, shame, and rage, reside.[3] Jung believed that a comprehensive understanding of these elements, along with the archetypes within the collective unconscious, facilitates a process known as individuation. This process entails embracing all facets of your personality, even those within your shadow, to promote personal growth and self-awareness.[4]

Dr. Jordan B. Peterson, a contemporary psychologist and scholar, has delved into Jungian psychology and its application to our modern understanding of the human psyche. In particular, he has explored the concept of the monster within the context of Jungian theory.[5] Drawing on Dr. Jung's foundation, Dr. Peterson considers the monster an embodiment of what Jungians call the shadow. The monster is a symbolic representation of these shadow elements, representing our inner struggles, our capacity for malice, and the potential for chaos.[6] Like Dr. Jung, Dr. Peterson believes confronting and integrating the monster—acknowledging our monstrous aspects—is essential for personal growth and individuation.[7] He emphasizes that facing inner demons is a fundamental step toward self-realization and psychological well-being.

By exploring the monster within the framework of Jungian theory, Peterson offers a contemporary lens through which we can better understand our human complexities and the transformative journey of embracing our shadows to become more fully realized individuals. As we move through the rest of my story, I will refer to the persona, shadow, and monster, as well as post-traumatic stress injury and moral injury.

Post-Traumatic Stress Injury

It is my opinion, and it is becoming widely accepted, that post-traumatic stress is not a disorder, nor is it a mental health issue. It is an injury, a neurological issue.[8] There are mental health issues that are associated with PTS, and they present as symptoms such as depression and anxiety; however, the neurological issues with PTS rest in the amygdala. Fight or flight, hypervigilance, sleep disturbances, cognitive function, and compassion fatigue are psychological changes that cannot be compelled. These are automatic and normal human responses to stressors and trauma.[9] This mechanism drives survival. This is a cause and effect; therefore, I believe it is not a disorder or dysfunction but a normal response to negative stimuli.

Trauma is relative to the person experiencing it. It is deeply personal, and reactions to trauma are based on several factors, most importantly, the capacity of the person who is experiencing it to process the trauma. There is no requisite number or specific types of events that qualify. Each person has a limit. It is neither my right nor my business to judge where that limit may be.

Moral Injury

Moral injury shares similarities with post-traumatic stress, both stemming from life-threatening events with guilt and shame as core features.[10] Betrayal and loss of trust, common in moral injury, also characterize PTS. Notably, PTS includes hyperarousal, which is distinguished from moral injury. One can experience moral injury without meeting PTS criteria, and distress from moral events may yield different symptoms than fear-based traumatic events.[11]

In the face of challenging circumstances, moral injury can emerge when individuals act in ways that contradict their deeply held moral beliefs or witness events that conflict with those values.[12] This can lead to a wide range of distress, including psychological, behavioral, social, and spiritual. The key reactions to moral injury are guilt, shame, disgust, anger, and an inability to self-forgive. Guilt is a form of distress that arises from a morally injurious act, while shame extends to a negative self-perception and cognitive distortion. Disgust and anger may stem from perpetration or betrayal, and an inability to self-forgive can result in self-sabotaging behaviors.[13]

Core features of moral injury, such as guilt and shame, are associated with more severe PTS, depression, and functional impairment. Notably, events involving perpetration outside one's values are linked to increased re-experiencing, guilt, and self-blame compared to life-threatening traumatic events.[14] Nightmares, inexplicable human tragedy, and events leading to moral injury chip away at personal resilience and, at some point, if unchecked, will lead to experiencing an entire psychological breakdown.[15]

A Simple Marker and Indelible Mark

In late July 2020, I was assigned to a patrol services district in the northeast portion of the county. My designated area at the time was sprawling, so large that it bordered and co-existed with a university police department and two municipal departments. Interstate 75 split my zone. Heavy traffic flow and, by my estimation, state troopers spread too thin, leading to our frequent response to the interstate until a trooper arrived. They were indeed a welcome sight.

The day began as any other; it was hot enough to melt the polish on your boots and render your body armor rancid by the end of a shift. The morning passed with no excitement to speak of. It was nearly noon, and I contemplated lunch options as I traveled eastbound on one of the major east/west roadways that bracketed my area. A call came across my in-car radio as I tried to decide between eating the wrap or a healthier option already in the passenger seat. Dispatch relayed that a pickup truck lost control while merging into traffic on Interstate 75 northbound. I listened intently as more details were provided, and I accelerated and activated my emergency equipment. I knew, or at least I thought I was the closest one.

Our dispatcher voiced an additional update that a person had been ejected from the vehicle onto the shoulder and was being checked on by good Samaritans. This is never good. My gut turned, and I prayed, "God, don't do this to me." I arrived on the scene relatively quickly, surprised to see one of the traffic units and another deputy who happened to be in the area had arrived on the scene. They were approaching the truck,

Introduction

now at rest on all four wheels, facing southbound and well into the grassy shoulder of the interstate. Near the truck were two inconsolable teen boys. They did not appear injured, so I turned my attention to people gathered by the cattle fence about ten feet from the truck.

As I approached, I saw two sock-covered feet belonging to someone lying supine behind a tree. My jaw tightened, and I moved closer to see an off-duty nurse, who was a passerby, and another Samaritan performing CPR on what appeared to be a teenage girl. There was no visible physical trauma. Just then, fire rescue approached. They arrived just after I did. Luckily, the station is less than two miles from the crash site, and they had easy access to the on-ramp. The medics quickly assessed their young patient and relieved the nurse. As they took over, I turned my attention to the boys, clearly in shock but lucid enough to give a brief and fragmented account of their experience.

A panting and frantic boy said they got onto Interstate 75 and swerved to miss a car. The young driver overcorrected, sending the truck into a clockwise spin and rolling over onto the grass shoulder. The ruts on the right shoulder and in the grass and the damage to the truck confirmed their recollection. I found out later that the boy I was talking to was the driver, and the other boy was the young girl's brother. She had been sitting in the backseat, windows down, at the time of the rollover and was ejected. More medics arrived on the scene and checked on the boys, and I returned briefly to the young girl.

I was standing next to the fire captain when his medics pronounced the young girl dead on the scene. She was 17, slightly older than my daughter at the time. I looked at the captain and said, "I don't know how many more of these I have left in me." The captain, whose face was drawn and weathered

Introduction

by 33 years of firefighting, looked at me and replied, "I don't either." There was a pause as he looked through me, and without another word, the captain turned and walked away.

It was time to set priorities for work and assign tasks of scene preservation and information gathering while the troopers were en route. The deputies who beat me to the scene seemed overwhelmed, not by emotion, but by the perceived complexity of the scene. One of them was relatively new, just a few months solo on the job. We began working, and the troopers arrived on the scene. The troopers were taking photos of the scene and moving about like bees, intent and clear on their missions.

Now in charge of the investigation, the troopers asked one of us to stay with the girl until the medical examiner arrived, and then he disappeared as quickly as he had come. I looked at the younger deputy, my back to the now-gathering crowd; she looked beyond me and said she would stay with the girl if I would deal with her dad. Confused by her reply, I turned and saw a man crumbling emotionally and moving as quickly as he could toward his daughter, who was now lying under a white sheet.

His jaw was clenched so tightly that his face twisted; it was the look of indescribable pain. As he got closer, I think he realized at the same time I did that I was the only thing standing between him and his little girl. I had no idea what I was going to say or do. His little girl was gone, and there was nothing I could do or say to change that. I did know that were I in his position, what it would take to prevent me from getting to my little girl and that I would not be enough. To that point in my professional life, I had never been pushed, punched, kicked, or even touched by anyone who had the intent to harm me. I was able to de-escalate or physically end any confrontation

Introduction

before one began. But at that moment, I believed this man was going to beat my ass, and I was going to let him.

Note: The rest of the story from Indelible Mark should be here to complete the vignette and thought, along with the lesson I learned. My journey did not begin here and certainly does not end here.

Chapter 1

When it All Began

It is widely accepted that trauma experienced later in life and one's ability to mitigate the effects of trauma are influenced by adverse childhood experiences.[1] So, my journey begins here. I was raised by a loving mother and father, who, as I write this passage, have been married for more than 53 years. My sister, a scant ten months older, was a protective big sister. My parents struggled financially early on, as most young couples did. They traveled for work, bringing us to Tampa via Bradenton and Memphis, where I spent the first six years of my life. My father worked hard and traveled, meeting with customers to sell lumber and other building materials. At the time, I thought he sold stuff like 2x4s and plywood, only to find out later that he brokered the import and sale of cargo on container ships full of lumber from as far away as Malaysia and Singapore. I undersold my father when I was younger. My mother, a homemaker, mortgage broker, and bank executive, did the heavy lifting, keeping all of us in line.

When my father was home, quality time consisted of

watching old black-and-white war movies and the Black Sheep Squadron, and this was our time together. I had a box full of G.I. Joe action figures and knew each action figure's dossier and background story cold. I would daydream of the real-life adventures of the people that each action figure must have been modeled after. As a young boy, I would spend hours playing G.I. Joe or *playing guns outside*. My father would entertain my friends and me with stories of his days as a paratroopera *screaming eagle;* he is a patriot and proud of his service.

My parents were active in service and civic clubs, volunteering at children's homes and the Shriners Hospital. Patriotism and service were always front and center and valued heavily by my family. Military service was a family tradition going back as far as Hampton Roads. A well-developed sense of patriotism and service shaped who I was to become.

Friends and the Teen Years

My friend group was a tight group of neighborhood boys who, despite our diverging paths, still call my parents Mr. and Mrs. White to this day. As far as organized sports, I played T-ball and football, swam, and even tried my hand at wrestling. Swimming was the one that stuck and carried me through high school.

I was the runt of the litter. With a lean swimmer's physique and 6'1", I tipped the scales at 165 pounds, 167 soaking wet. I was lean and shredded, and my smile and dimples did little to increase my *street cred* as a *bruiser*. Luckily, I had my close friends, Jay, Robbie, and Wayne. Each of them was bigger and stronger than the next.

In line, they resembled an evolutionary chart of a *manchild*. Robbie was good-natured and gentle; Wayne was a physical monster but quiet and kind; and Jay was and remains a loyal and unhinged lunatic with a sense of adventure and no fear. No one messed with me, first because I was a good guy and second because tooth chippers surrounded me should the need arise. Luckily, that day never came. We were all brothers from another mother and could be found generally in each other's company.

I was not one of the popular kids, but I could be counted on to be consistent. What you saw was what you got. I was sensitive, empathetic, and despised bullies. When I was growing up, I was bullied by a bigger neighborhood kid. In that instance, it was more pushing and shoving, never a full-on fight. As a teen, I had no idea how I would fare in a fight. I had no idea if I could take a punch.

Luckily, I was slow to anger and only responded physically once during my teen years. A kid during my junior year thought he was tough. He was talking trash and said he was going to fight me. The entire school knew before I did. Peer pressure and ego demanded that I stand up for myself and face this kid. We were evenly matched by physical stature, but I had no reason to fight. But, if I did not fight, I would be painted as weak or an easy target for the next dude.

After school, I met the kid at the bus loading area. As he approached, I was surrounded. This indicated that he broadcasted his intent to beat me up to the entire school. As he squared off, I asked if he still wanted to fight me. He said yes and raised his hands. What came next was a blur. When the dust settled, I was untouched and unscathed. Everyone learned something that day. Words and actions have consequences, and I was not to be messed with. That was my first and last off-duty fight and the last time anyone picked on me.

I was a good kid and did not get into trouble or get caught.

My friends often dropped me off before wreaking havoc, knowing my parent's wrath would come if I were involved in their shenanigans.

The Guys

Robbie and I were very close. We were almost inseparable in our senior year. Nearly every weekend, I would stay at his house. Robbie had an older brother named Carson, our unofficial hero then. When Robbie and I met, Carson was much older, married, and out of the house. He worked for the municipal police department and guided us toward that path.

Wayne was the mediator and not usually down for shenanigans. He was the calm voice of reason. He was the conscience on your shoulder whispering sage advice so as not to get yourself *effed* up. Wayne was good at this and was a staple of Robbie's house.

Jay is another story. He was always ready for a fight should one spontaneously erupt. Jay was the driver. He had a large conversion van, like the A-Team van, but blue. He carted us all around in it whenever we went out.

Late in my senior year, I met Joel. Joel was the little brother of my then-girlfriend's friend. I must highlight the irony of using the word little to describe Joel. Though five years younger, he was physically a full-grown man at 13.

The friend group dwindled as life progressed. Robbie, my best man and best friend, passed away on June 13, 2018. We had not spoken for four years before his passing. Ego and a crossed boundary kept us apart. Wayne moved out of state, and Jay was contracting overseas or living on a mountain. We kept in touch over the years and even saw each other from time to time.

Despite the age gap, Joel would be one that grew with me over the years and became a sounding board for many of the pages you are about to read. Other friends from my childhood did not make this journey with me. My path was narrow. I did my best to make the right decisions and, early on, divested myself of those who were either incapable or unwilling to change.

Grown Up Decisions

I knew I wanted to serve in the military but was unsure which branch. Initially, I was all Army. I went and sat down with the recruiter, and he, of course, promised the world. *Eleven bang-bang* (Infantry specialty of 11-B) with Airborne and Ranger *options* were thrown my way. I am unsure today, and I was less sure then that these *options* were real or just part of a recruiting tool for overzealous teens.

Then, I met with the Air Force recruiter. He was a mild-mannered man, and his job before recruiting duty was as an air traffic controller. He listened to my desires, merged my wide-eyed dreams with his profession, and told me about the wonderful world of the Combat Controller. I was convinced the scarlet beret would be mine. I had the recruiting pamphlets, posters, and VHS tapes. The whole deal. He drove me to MacDill to meet with controllers and PJs who were doing pre-screening and preparing enlistees by giving specific workouts and conducting the physical fitness evaluations before a recruiter allowed a potential recruit to sign on the straight-solid line. I was lean, physically strong, and more important than that, I could swim.

I passed the pre-screening and went to the military entrance processing stations (MEPS). Everything was going well for me until the eye test. I have little to no low-light depth perception, a critical ability for landing planes and calling in air strikes. So, plan B. My recruiter assured me that signing an open general contract would be suitable, and I could pick a job later. I could ship off to basic training as soon as I graduated in June 1992.

During the latter half of my senior year, *love* got in the way of those plans. I met a nice girl, and she was the cheer captain. That's a big deal if you're in high school. As time grew near, I grew anxious. In response to my hormones overriding any sense of discipline, I withdrew from the delayed enlistment program in late May, just before graduation. In hindsight, this saved me from an open general contract.

Despite having a summer girlfriend and solid buddies, I was aimless for months. Robbie enlisted in the Marine Corps in the Fall of 1992 and went to Parris Island. My girlfriend broke up with me, and roughly four months later, I traveled to the Island to see Robbie graduate from boot camp. It was one of the most impressive things I had witnessed, and I was so envious of his accomplishment. Moreover, I was completely overwhelmed by the level of pride I had because he was my friend and now a Marine.

We left the Island, and Robbie stayed behind to report to Marine Combat Training (MCT) to train as a light mortarman, 0341. After MCT, Robbie came home on leave, and we went to a seedy tattoo parlor so he could get the Eagle, Globe, and Anchor tattooed on his left bicep. He earned his *club* patch, so why not? Man, his mom, who is 5' tall with heels, was pissed! After she cried, she moved the step stool over to Robbie and broke him off a fresh one: five fingers and a whole hand across the face.

Robbie was selected out of MCT for a special duty

assignment. After his leave, Robbie reported to his permanent duty station, the Marine Corps Barracks, Washington, D.C., 8th, and I. Robbie had been selected for the Silent Drill Platoon. It was time for me to get to work. I was committed. I had to go to the recruiter and enlist.

Chapter 2

Off We Go, Into the Wild Blue Yonder

"I [state your full name], Do solemnly swear that I will support and defend the Constitution of the United States against all enemies, foreign and domestic; that I will bear true faith and allegiance to the same; and that I will obey the orders of the President of the United States and the orders of the officers appointed over me, according to regulations and the Uniform Code of Military Justice. So help me God."

— *The Oath of Enlistment*

The day Robbie went to Washington, D.C., I was searching for my G.I. Joe adventure. I went to the Air Force recruiter the day Robbie left. Luckily, all my paperwork was intact and sitting in his filing cabinet. MEPS followed later in the week. I was still in great shape. Although I could not be a controller, I could still serve in any other enlisted specialty without a depth perception requirement. Now, with a little more maturity, I weighed my decisions against what I wanted to do when and if I separated. I still wanted a story, but it needed to be practical if I decided not to stay twenty years.

Prospects for jobs that sounded sexy to me then were limited in the Air Force. My choices were Explosive Ordnance Disposal (EOD), rotor wing crew chief, B52 tail gunner, Survival Specialist, and Security Police. I recall my father telling me jokingly before going to MEPS that he had received dozens of calls since 1965, wanting him to jump out of planes and kill people. Dad was not very subtle, and I knew I needed to choose a path that would suit me in the civilian world. I wanted to go into law enforcement, so the next natural step was Security Police. I signed up for the delayed enlistment program in May of 1993 and was going to ship on 48 hours' notice.

By Monday, May 17, 1993, I was on a plane to San Antonio to begin my four-year journey that would last more than fourteen years. I arrived in San Antonio late at night and was shuttled to Lackland Air Force Base, my first time away from home, family, and friends. I recall the night being a whirlwind. I finally got in my bunk at about 0200 hours, twenty hours after my trip began. The following day began as they would for the next four months. Early, with heavy doses of screaming and attention to detail.

Fire Watch and A Change

As we move through the several stages of life, we search for who we will become—borrowing traits from peer groups, our culture, music, and other influences. As we exit high school, we look for our first adult persona and will likely identify with the most significant influence on us. This is nothing more than what I imagine would be described as *branding* today. At that time, nothing was more influential to me than military service. I was raised with a solid moral compass and traditional values, so off I went, a deep dive into being an Airman. I felt that service was a worthy purpose; this would be my brand for the foreseeable future.

Each recruit in basic training gets several opportunities at Fire Watch or Dorm Guard. It's the same job, but Fire Watch makes it sound more harrowing. The Dorm Guard stood at the dormitory door for two hours per shift while everyone slept. Rare disturbances occurred, and staying awake after training in the Texas heat was challenging. I was Dorm Guard several times in training, but one shift sticks out.

This shift sticks in my head as I experienced one of those *before and after* events that mark time in your life. Standing at the door of the 322nd Basic Military Training Squadron's Flight 312, Dorm A3, I was standing alone, facing a full-length mirror just inside and to the right of the entryway. I looked at my reflection and did not recognize myself. I seemed older somehow, focused, committed, and clear. This was when it all clicked. I saw the man I could become, and I never looked back.

I completed basic training and moved to the other side of Lackland to my new home, Building 10253, the Security Police dormitory. I completed the student leadership course, machine gunner's qualification, the security police academy, and basic ground combat or air base ground defense courses, earning my badge and blue beret.

The Pacific Northwest

Being from Central Florida, I selected all Florida-based installations on my assignment dream sheet. My first choice was MacDill in Tampa, but the Air Force's first choice was

McChord in Tacoma. Rain, snow, grunge music, and Mt. Rainier would be staples for the next four years.

I qualified as a security specialist, which was my specialty, but I was fortunate enough that some security troops were also cross-trained and certified for law enforcement duties. Once we qualified for our primary duties, we were selected to work the entry control points. After qualifying at the gates, we were moved into patrol. The streets of McChord would be my training grounds, and I loved every second of it.

The Body

My first encounter with death would come in 1994, when an Airman in my squadron, my former next-door neighbor, got into legal trouble. It was unclear what he did, but it triggered a lengthy investigation. He was confined to barracks, and shortly after, he went missing. He had been missing for a few days, and no one had seen or heard from him. A few days later, while on patrol, my roommate found the body. The location where his body was recovered would be my first crime scene.

He was in his green Jeep, backed into the woods off a trail in the base's south forty. The Jeep was now out of gas and cold to the touch. The Airman was in the driver's seat, slumped over, with a congealed drip of blood coming from his head. The Jeep and the Airman had been there for a couple of days.

I was twenty years old, and this was my first dead body. I never knew what the issue was, and my roommate and I never talked about it after. My roommate, however, was the lead singer of a well-known local band and wrote a song, "The Body." This was his way of expressing his experience and was written but not performed until he left active duty.

There was no mechanism in place for counseling or

debriefing after such a call. The choices were to drive on or be placed on the *rubber gun squad* and have your clearance and status pulled. In short, suck it up and drive on. In retrospect, I believe this was my first exposure to trauma.

An Early Lesson?

In April 1995, I met a blonde-haired country girl who had been assigned to McChord. After a short courtship, I proposed on the beach. We were married in December 1995. However, a series of unfortunate events led me to dissolve our partnership and go our separate ways. The new plan was to separate from the Air Force on May 17, 1997, enter the Air Force Reserve, leave, and return to Tampa to work.

I was in a loveless marriage to a woman who destroyed me through cruelty and infidelity. Transitioning from the military to civilian workforce while moving across the country with no soft landing afforded by an awaiting job would be a heavy lift for a 23-year-old. I only had half a plan at best, and there was no plan B.

With the benefit of time and distance, I realized that we were both young. The greatest lesson I learned was that I would never settle for anything again, and I knew what love should look like, or at least what it did not look like.

Chapter 3

A Rebuilding Season

This rebuilding season was formative in my life. I transitioned from active duty into the civilian world while navigating a divorce and searching for a new career. During the summer of 1997, I worked a retail security job, took college classes, attended the police academy, and passed the state law enforcement officer exam to occupy my time. I even dated a bit, but nothing serious.

Emotionally, this wasn't easy, and I had to be conscious of my habits. My friends were spending time in bars drinking, and the last thing I needed was to try and drown my sorrows. Self-medicating was not the answer. There are no answers in bottles. As the son of an alcoholic, my father has been in recovery for forty years; I am fully aware of what addiction brings. I was conscious not to overdo it and never drank out of depression or boredom. I knew I needed purpose and had to get on track or be lost.

Getting yourself sorted out sends a message that you have something to offer and the capacity for more. This is when I met Michelle. At the time, she worked full-time at a small hometown law office, worked weekends as a waitress, and was enrolled full-time in college on an academic scholarship. She was driven, and after weeks of relentless pursuit and a *test* date with her and her guy friends in Ybor City, we finally had our first date on November 19, 1997.

I knew by early December that she was the one. I had never felt anything so strongly in my life. I would see flashes of light and get butterflies when she was around. She was beautiful, and she was everything right with the world. I needed to get off my ass and make something happen before I was left behind.

Plan A

Anyone in the first responder and military communities knows that anything requiring paperwork rarely happens quickly. There was a waiting list, and there was no easy way to be hired by the organization where I eventually worked. I did not apply to other agencies; this was the second half of the plan. I would be a deputy for a large law enforcement agency in central Florida.

I completed my new hire packet for the sheriff's office, and during the process, I was offered a chance to be a reserve deputy. Reserve deputies are certified deputies but do not get paid. I accepted the opportunity gleefully, but I needed to pay my bills. I did not know how long the wait for the reserve position would be or how long it would be for a full-time position to be offered. I worked in retail then, and although being paid commission and free clothing was a plus, it did not serve me. I needed to reframe my mindset and return to something more my speed.

Off We Go Again

I needed discipline and bearing. I was still serving in the active Air Force Reserve and had been newly assigned to the 919th Special Operations Wing at Duke Field, also known as Eglin Field #3, Florida. In November and early December of 1997, I took every opportunity to work on individual orders because it paid better than retail and was much more fulfilling. The 919th was an interesting experience, providing me with access to the special operations aircraft platforms used by the Air Force. Driving four hours on the weekends for a couple of workdays would get old quickly, so I needed a closer unit.

As fortune would have it, I met a master sergeant at the 919th. More importantly to this story, this master sergeant was also a government employee at Headquarters U.S. Special Operations Command (SOCOM) at MacDill in Tampa—just a 23-mile commute from my front door. It was also an active-duty major command augmented by reservists on long, continuous orders. On my birthday, the master sergeant told me there was an E5 billet open at SOCOM for the Joint Elite Guard Force, a prestigious and highly sought-after position. He explained that the position requires that you be a minimum of E4, eligible for E5, and pass an in-person interview with the operation's superintendent and Provost Marshall.

A Whole New Level

With a fresh, high-and-tight haircut and always polished boots, I met with the operation's superintendent, a Chief Master Sergeant. I must have channeled my inner *Hooah*, and he offered me the position on the spot. I could not even process the information before my photo was taken for my credentials. I was placed on orders and reported shortly after. Thank you for the opportunity, Rusty.

I shared the news with Michelle, and she was excited for me. I now had a full-time job with benefits, at least for the next 180 days, my training, and my annual tour. Theoretically, I could have been employed eight months out of the year before I needed to find waivers.

I reported to duty on my first day in December 1997. The guard force was a joint services detachment within the command's Security Management Office, combining Marine and Army military police, Navy masters at arms, and Air Force Security Forces. I was working with hand-selected professionals, performing physical security for a major command filled with my time's most capable warriors and enablers. The officers and NCOs I met in those early days and the men I served with post-9/11 left an indelible mark.

A Welcomed Call

In early January 1998, I received a call from the recruitment and screening section at the Sheriff's Office. They informed me that they were building a Reserve I class and wanted to add me to the list. The Reserve Academy would begin in February, and classes would be from 1800 to 2200 hours Monday through Thursday and last eleven weeks.

Michelle was my first call, and then I informed the command of the opportunity, and they moved me to the dayshift to accommodate my class hours. From February to May 1998, I worked a Panama schedule (Monday/Tuesday, Friday/Saturday/Sunday, Wednesday/Thursday. rotating weekly) at the command from 0600-1700 and Monday through Thursday nights from 1800-2200 hours at the academy. This schedule was physically and mentally demanding. It required me on duty and class days to leave my house at 0500, return home around 2230 hours, and repeat for eleven weeks.

Two Uniforms

I began the Reserve Academy and met my classmates. This may sound dismissive, but only one classmate played a significant role in my life and is present today. I sat in the back row on the aisle, and to my immediate left sat Richard G. Over the next 25 years and five months, Rich and I would be each other's defensive tactics partner, handcuffing dummy, zone partner, groomsman, and most importantly, friend. Rich and I began our careers together.

Chapter 4

The Office

May 19, 1998, on the eve of my first shift as a civilian law enforcement officer, I watched a story unfold which ended with the deaths of a child, three law enforcement officers, and the piece of shit responsible for it all. Detective Randy Bell and Ricky Childers of the Tampa Police Department were investigating the fatal shooting of a young boy.

The person of interest was taken into custody for questioning. During the transport by Detectives Bell and Childers, the subject was able to free his hands using a concealed handcuff key and wrestled away one of the detective's firearms. He was able to kill both detectives and retrieve his SKS-style rifle from the trunk. The suspect fled on Interstate 75 when Florida Highway Patrol Trooper James Crooks stopped him. The suspect fired on the trooper, killing him. The suspect barricaded himself in a gas station and eventually succumbed to the effects of bullets.

Undeterred and with purpose, I reported to District III the following day for roll call. I introduced myself to the sergeant, who looked at me and handed me a black mourning band to place over my star. On my first day of duty, my star was draped in a mourning band. I quickly learned that this five-pointed star would be the heaviest piece of metal I would ever carry. However, it would be years before I fully realized how heavy it could get.

I met my field training officer, Gary, a very senior deputy with the patience of Job and the cool of Billy D. (Star Wars-Lando Calrissian, *the younger crowd*); Gary was great and took his time to train me. I wrote several reports with Gary and learned a lot of *old-guy stuff*. He never said anything to the effect of *forgetting everything you learned; this is how we do it out here*. He was encouraging and practical.

10-51, Enroute

On day four of reserve field training, I was writing a report for a runaway juvenile. A message queued up on the mobile data terminal screen. In green letters on a black screen, it said something about having your rookie call recruitment and screening. I picked up my large Erickson cell phone and called right away. The detective on the other end of the phone asked if I wanted to get paid to be a deputy. I was ecstatic, and he instructed me to come to sign the paperwork to become a full-time, duly sworn sheriff's deputy. I hung up and excitedly told Gary the news. Thoroughly unimpressed, Gary lit his cigarette and said, "Not until you finish that report."

Later that day, I signed the paperwork and was given my new badge number (PID) and a start date of July 13, 1998. I called Michelle and my parents to tell them the news. Then I called Robbie, who had also applied for a full-time position when I applied for a Reserve One position and a full-time position. Robbie told me he got the call and started on July 13, too. I was assigned a Personnel Identification Number, also called a PID, 4569; he was 4574. Wide-eyed, full of potential, and eager, a new brand-Deputy White was born.

Michelle had big aspirations and was working hard on her future. I desperately wanted to be a part of it. Through the normal progression of relationships, Michelle and I grew closer. I felt complete with her and that we could meet any challenge no matter what the future holds. I asked Michelle to marry me, and she accepted. We were married on July 8, 2000.

The Rookie

My purpose was clear: through tireless dedication, I wanted to be the best I could be, set the standard, serve the profession faithfully, and protect those who could not protect themselves. These were my expectations for my actions, ultimately meeting my obligations to the organization. I was on my path, and my usefulness to the profession and the organization throughout my career would measure my success. Nowhere in my definition of success was rank, title, or position. I remained loyal to my purpose, and over the years, I excelled in every professional venture.

At the time, the prevailing professional culture ranked new personnel in an unofficial hierarchy. Like troops of apes or herds of wild animals, your toughness or prowess ranked you in this society—professional bearing, the ability to effectively and efficiently dole out measured violence when needed, stoicism in the face of danger, and the ability to remain emotionless and calm in the most harrowing circumstances were the marks you were rated on. If I wanted to be counted among this troop's top echelon and to survive and thrive, I would need to build my brand as a *tooth-chipping* enforcer, a meat eater. In other words, don't act like food if you don't want to be eaten.

To this end, I built a technical knowledge base to solve nearly any problem. I had a knack for planning and problem-solving in rapidly cascading situations. I enjoyed anticipating problems, mitigating them by flipping switches, and staying one step ahead. I refined my ability to look at a scene or situation and devise a tactical plan, set work priorities, and communicate the information while driving to a scene. This came as natural to me as blinking. I thrived in chaos and had a *one-liner* for every situation.

Although I initially had a baby face, I had finally grown into my adult body. Now, 6' 1" and 220 pounds, my naturally peaked eyebrows gave the permanent appearance of a scowl, my haircut was high and tight, and I was all business. Highly pressed and shined, I often went home on meal break to starch and re-press my shirt before returning to the second half of the shift.

I wore black leather and Kevlar-lined gloves to prevent needle sticks, sharps, or being punctured by barbs on chain link fences. These gloves went on before every call in which I may be expected to touch someone. In time, my gloves became a queue to local bar patrons that I was not there for the pretzels and served as a sign to deputies that I was there to work.

A professional bearing and command presence in uniform is necessary and will diffuse most physical or verbal confrontations. My zone partners thought this was witchcraft rather than an attribute, but my presence brought order. Carry yourself as if you came to do business; those less committed will shrink when you walk in the door. Those committed to silliness got to play *Choose Your Adventure* or *FAFO~Fuck Around and Find Out*.

It was not until much later, near the end of my career, that I realized that all of the risk-taking behaviors that fueled this persona building, this branding of the shaved-head unflappable hard charger, was important to the foundation but only worked to a point. The adage, what got you here won't get you there slowly approached. Eventually, I would have to rebrand myself to be a *company man*. The only difference between the former and the latter was the purchase of a comb and hair gel. I simply changed my physical appearance.

Chapter 5

September 11, 2001

Being assigned to Headquarters U. S. Special Operations Command and having the opportunity to be associated with the people that comprised the special operations forces enterprise was a great honor. I was invited to reenlist and remain with the command in 2001, and on September 4, 2001, I reenlisted for six more years. This reenlistment was a pivotal moment in my story. Without it, I would have separated with an honorable discharge at midnight, September 10, 2001.

On September 11, 2001, I was asleep and scheduled to report for my shift at the sheriff's office at 1300 hours when my mother called me just before 0900 and told me to turn on the news. I turned to the news just moments before Flight 157 crashed into the World Trade Center's South Tower. Although the probability is nearly nil, one crash may be an accident, but two? It was obvious that this was an intentional act.

I immediately called the command. I could barely get out my full name before I was ordered to report the next morning at 0500 hours. The urgency in their voice was unmistakable, and I reported for duty at the office that day as scheduled. It would be my last shift for the foreseeable future.

The following day, arriving at the main gate, I immediately noticed the traffic. 100% identification and vehicle checks were being conducted. There were no trucks or buses. It was hard to miss the HMMV with a mounted M2 .50 caliber machine gun facing northbound on Dale Mabry Highway. All other gates were closed. It was a mess, but the base cops were managing well.

I arrived at the command early, hoping to beat traffic and get an early jump on any information or a vague picture of the way forward. The command was buzzing around the clock for the next several months. Bollards and barricades were operational and staffed. We needed more bodies if we were going to sustain this tempo for the foreseeable future. Reservists, Air National Guard, and Army National Guard were mobilized to backfill and augment active units. That's someone else's story.

We all knew there would be an active duty recall if we went to war; we did not know when that might be. I was proactive and initially volunteered for six-month orders, but by December 1, 2001, Title 10 would have me for another year. Then another, and then some. In total, my post-9/11 commitment lasted 37 months and 18 days.

The men I served with heavily influenced my growth and maturity. They each served as the benchmark for professionalism, warriors, leadership, friendship, and loyalty. The 37 months after 9/11 would become an important plot point of my hero's journey. Being associated with these men during this time was a great source of pride and, later, my greatest frustration.

In the months following 9/11, the larger command

concentrated on operations in Afghanistan while meeting its other global commitments. The guard force concentrated on physical security and force protection, translating to long hours and months of straight-through work. We had what remained of the original cast, but additional personnel were added to the guard force. We also had a few soldiers, Rangers, who were reassigned from the commandant's office. They were a welcomed addition and would grow with us in time.

Initially, these characters would join me in providing physical security for the command and its facilities. Then, the Secretary of Defense ordered that each combatant commander have a personal protective detail. By Secretary Rumsfeld's order, the command's security management office (SMO) began building its own protective security detachment, or PSD.

The early days of PSD were exciting. We were established with the kit we had on hand at the command, specifically what the guard force had in the armory. Although this would suffice initially, we knew we would have to grow to support the mission properly.

The generals and admirals who held the position did not seem to mind our existence and saw us as necessary to meet the directive. In the early days, we worked on doctrine and managed with the personnel already assigned to the SMO. The commander we had at the time mainly traveled to Europe, around town, and the capital region. So, for this boss, the home team was suitable. He tended to use us more as valets or junior aides de camp. I think he missed the point. However, he soon retired, and we were blessed with General Bryan (Doug) Brown, who was previously the command's deputy commander.

By this point, GWOT, the Global War on Terror, was in

full swing, and General Brown knew that we would be necessary and had been underutilized. He was much busier than the previous boss, very personable, and funnier than the other guy.

General Brown would travel to any place Special Operations Forces (SOF) was located, including Central Command's area of operations, South America, the Pacific, and even a mountaintop forward operating base (FOB) in Afghanistan. He was an incredible leader—a warrior poet, brilliant, decisive, and undeniably competent. The team believed we would have to remove him physically if there was an issue. We figured he would be more inclined to stick around and fight it out with us than to be evacuated.

In the beginning, the home team covered him everywhere except in theater. This would soon change. It was explained that General Brown was downrange and noticed familiar faces; we did not surround him, but SOF elements were already in the country and reassigned as PSD. He knew these people should be engaged otherwise were it not for his presence. At the time, in-country SOF elements would be diverted from their missions and assigned as his PSD. The larger force also practiced this, pulled special operations elements away from their intended use, and assigned PSD duties to provisional dignitaries.

One day, General Brown called us into his office. He wanted to see exactly how many people he had assigned to PSD and how many people it took to support just him when he traveled. Soon after this meeting, the home team got some ringers.

Operators due for a headquarters or staff tour were assigned to headquarters, supporting PSD and doing various jobs within their skill sets. New team leadership was soon on board. Senior enlisted operators, E8s and E9s (Master Sergeants and Sergeants Major), from the various numbered teams and or colored task forces, *Quiet Professionals*, the type that could grow a beard before lunch, joined the team, and it was off to the races.

To be clear, I was not an *operator*, but they did not care; we were trusted members of the team. Rank existed only to remind the Defense Finance and Accounting Service what we got paid on the first and fifteenth. Everyone contributed and was relied upon for their strengths. Any shortfalls were shored up with training or mentorship. This new world included running hot ranges, safety briefs like *If you shoot me, I'll shoot you back,* and the type of leadership and self-ownership on a level that has been unmatched in any of my experiences. Each of my teammates was humble and would only admit that they just did their best to do *their share of the work*. I learned more about leadership, warriors, loyalty, and what the word teammate meant from these men.

This was it. I was surrounded by the most professional warriors on the planet and in a position to work directly with them—an opportunity to do my best to do my share. We would be the bubble surrounding the boss wherever he went. I took part in dozens of trips within the continental U.S., or CONUS planned and executed without issues. Planning, executing, and solving problems on the fly became instinctive; we were a well-oiled machine. Living out of bags and moving from one place to the next was part of the job.

Our days began routinely with PT, and we would work out and run. At the time, I was a big kid. My run pace may have been a shuffle, but I could push your car where it needed to go if you ran out of gas. I routinely carried one of my more playful teammates around the office on my back as he was trying to apply a standing rear naked choke while telling me to go to sleep. Slinging heavy weights allowed me to reach a body weight of 240 pounds. I was under the body fat limit for my age and height but still big enough for at least one person to take cover behind me.

At this point, I was built for breaking shit, and I started with my ankle. Yes, I broke my ankle playing a rough game of *zoo ball* with some teammates. I pressed on through the duty day, and the chief walked into the office late in the afternoon and saw my leg propped up. My foot looked like a purple cartoon balloon. He asked what the doctor said and was surprised when I told him I had not seen him yet. The following morning, I reported to the clinic as ordered. My ankle was indeed broken, and there was some suspicion about ligament damage as well. I argued with the doctor over a cast, and we compromised on a walking boot. The boot was ineffective, and after about six weeks, the decision was made to put me in a cast. This single game of *zoo ball* would begin nearly a year of surgeries and healing.

Shortly after my injury, opportunities for the team to go down range finally presented themselves, and the team took full advantage of them. My injury and the resulting surgeries prevented me from going down range with the team. I was relegated to gear, logistics, country clearances, etcetera, just admin and assorted hooah (little h). I missed the trips to Iraq, Asia, Afghanistan, Pakistan, and Eastern Europe. Between surgeries and castings, I would get the opportunity to run local missions and CONUS stuff, enough to make me feel like I was contributing, but not where I felt it mattered.

I healed and continued until my orders ended in November

2004, when I returned to the Sheriff's Office. In the end, supporting the *boss* and my teammates downrange, where I felt it made a difference, was not in the cards. My teammates, a tribe of the most extraordinary men I would have ever been associated with, served and smashed against the anvil of war. Breaking or broken, they returned with stories and scores of photos without me. I left with shame and regret, unfulfilled and empty. I fully embraced imposter syndrome.

For clarification, I was not upset that *I did not get to go to war*. I was upset because I let my teammates down. That is where I felt I needed to be, with my teammates, to serve when and where it mattered, and I was not. For years, I never said a thing to anyone because I was so ashamed and felt guilty that I was not there when it counted, that what I believed was my purpose on this planet had not been fulfilled.

In the years following my return to the sheriff's office, I returned to the command several times to complete my minimum annual obligations. By then, new faces were replacing the old faces, and they were doing business differently. The team I knew was gone, along with my opportunity to do my share. In September 2007, after nearly fourteen and a half years and a decade at the command, I quietly separated with an honorable discharge. Despite my achievements and commendations, I did not feel I had earned the right to be counted among my teammates.

I stayed in touch with most of the team, the ones with whom I was closest. In the years following, we would meet and tell old stories as if it were the first time we had heard them. The stories were always told the same way; if you were a douche when it happened, you were a douche when it was retold. I was in many stories but rarely felt like I rated their company. I felt like a little brother hanging out with his big brother and friends. They never treated me any differently, but I knew. I held onto this secret for fifteen years. I thought guilt and shame would fade or turn into something else. I thought I could outpace the feeling and atone for my shortfall by excelling elsewhere to prove that I rated. Nothing filled the hole.

Chapter 6

Back at the Office

In 2004, Michelle and I decided to try to have a baby. Despite Michelle being a baby whisperer, I was very apprehensive about the idea. I tried to justify my apprehension because I was still on active duty, and the future was uncertain regarding more orders or a return to the office. In all honesty, I was self-involved, although I did not admit it aloud. It was certain that Michelle wanted a baby, so we tried. In December 2004, our little girl was born one month after I returned to the office. Just over two years later, in early 2007, our son was born. We were now a family of four.

My active-duty orders ended on October 30, 2004, and I returned to the office the following Monday. I was the first person from the office to be mobilized because of the September 11th attacks. I was mobilized for thirty-seven months and eighteen days, making it the most extended deployment away from the office. With my wartime purpose unfulfilled, I knew that when I returned, I would have to double down, make up for lost time, and ensure that I continued to set myself apart from my peers. I needed to reaffirm my position in the district, so I hit the ground running.

I returned with more than three years of novel experience and exposure to outstanding leaders. Some specialty courses and insight into the process of higher-level decision-making provided me with a robust toolkit that served me for the rest of my career. While at the command, I became adept at planning and emergency management, mitigation, and problem-solving. I used my time convalescing to take as many FEMA and emergency management courses as possible. By the time I returned to the Office, I had amassed twenty-seven complete courses and had completed the entire professional development series. I was quite a nerd.

The week before returning to the office, I attended a weapons of mass destruction awareness course hosted by the Department of Homeland Security. It was a train-the-trainer course, and upon completion, I was qualified as a national WMD Awareness Course Instructor. Unfortunately, this was a tiny and selective niche in law enforcement at the time. Fortunately, I was one of three people in the organization with this skill set and the only one who could teach it.

I found teaching and instructing a passion that I became particularly good at. Watching recruits and responders from other disciplines experience their *aha* moments was fulfilling. I was driven and looking for an opportunity to instruct. In 2005, I was temporarily brought into the training unit to teach the newly developed Active Shooter training. I was asked to establish incident command system training regarding active shooter responses. This was the first solo instruction I would do at the office, and it was delivered to the entire command staff. I killed it, and my performance was directly responsible for my assignment to the newly formed Training Division.

Later, in this capacity, I would roll out all mandatory incident command system (ICS) training and training for issued personal protective equipment. I would also ensure compliance with the National Incident Management System (NIMS) by the 2007 deadline. I stood alone as the ICS and WMD guy at the top of the instructor heap. Not to remain stagnant, I was aware that, at the time, 85% of all terror attacks were carried out with explosives. I could not consider myself a practitioner if I missed 85% of the game. Luckily, the answer soon presented itself.

The Bomb Disposal Team-Initial Success, or Total Failure

The bomb squad was a coveted position with seven members. The squad required a year and a half of service on the team learning the procedures and equipment before applying for a class date to attend the FBI Hazardous Devices School at the United States Army Ordnance Munitions and Electronic Maintenance School. After that, you were required to serve five years on the team. Historically, guys on the team only left when they retired.

Luckily, the NIMS compliance came with team typing and set forth requirements for size, equipment, and duties. The office was the biggest game in town and had to be a type 1 team requiring ten technicians. One guy just retired from the team, so four new technicians must be added and trained before the 2007 deadline. This would be the first tryout for the team in my seven-year tenure at the office.

The tryouts were a grind; July in central Florida saw to it. A physical fitness evaluation began on the first day, followed by shooting qualifications. The second day was nothing but practical evaluations. You were given several specific tasks of mobility and agility while in the bomb suit and then later in chemical protective clothing with a respirator in the bomb suit. Bomb suits have no air conditioning, and most of the applicants were smoked and ineffective after the first portion of day two. Successful completion of the tryouts included the ability to follow very detailed instructions and then document your actions in the after-action report. The third day was an oral interview with the leaders of the regional bomb squad commanders.

After being selected, I became an active member of the team. I would spend the next year attending training courses, taking turns fetching gear with the other new guys, and getting the trucks for callouts or details. I waited a year for a class date and then got my class date. Michelle was four months pregnant with our son, and I was determined to be back well before our daughter's second birthday.

I attended the six-week residence course at Redstone Arsenal, Alabama. Again, this was a serious course; the year-to-year-and-a-half wait was to ensure you were prepared to attend the school. A test was given on the first day. There were no second chances. If you failed, you were packed and sent home. In this line of work, you need to be right the first time, every time. Hence, the motto, *'Initial Success or Total Failure,'* which underscores the high stakes and the need for precision in our work.

The course and the late summer heat in Alabama were challenging. I had an unmarked car for the course, and Huntsville is ninety miles from Nashville. I could take weekend flights home for less than $100 round trip, and I went home every weekend but one. On the weekdays, I could visit Michelle and our daughter via webcam each night.

I completed the course and became a bomb tech in training. My tenure on the bomb squad and my ability to teach emergency management and terrorism courses led to my being contracted to teach for the Department of Homeland Security and deliver courses nationally. Soon, I would be the ICS, WMD, and bomb guy.

I was a certified technician until December 2012. I made the long walk on dozens of calls. I had all successful disruptions and a successful hand entry. I had successful post-blast investigations, which led to convictions for making and placing destructive devices. I was trained as an explosive breacher and a HAZMAT technician. I had checked all of the boxes.

I was wholly dedicated to my professional roles, to such a degree that my roles as father and husband had been sacrificed. I thought my dedication was for the greater good, leading me closer to fulfilling my purpose. Leaving family functions for callouts was not a rare occasion. Professionally, time away impacted my duties as a field trainer and interfered with my ability to take on new assignments. It pulled me away from my duties as a newly promoted corporal. I was worried about missing opportunities to serve in other areas, cornering myself into the specialty team role. I did not want to make a career mistake by staying too long. So, I went to my boss. He was a major and had been on the SWAT team for much of his career, at every rank, and was now the commander as a major. After a short conversation about my future, he told me I had missed several opportunities. He concluded with a simple illustration and said I could be the corporal who had been on the bomb team for 25 years or the major who used to be on the bomb team. The decision was mine.

The conversation with the major and his confident answer fit my newfound ambition and healthy ego. After a discussion with the team, I resigned to pursue my career path as a supervisor. I was unsure if this was the right decision. Still, I believed I would be of more service in a leadership position moving forward rather than on a specialty team. It was time to move forward.

To this point, I had used over-commitment to avoid or drown the stress and sought more professional roles and responsibilities, hoping to keep myself busy and, on some level, fulfilled. I knew that I was spread thin physically and emotionally. I was having trouble sleeping, nightmares visited me regularly, and I just wanted to be alone when I was not working. I had no idea what was happening to me. Still, there was no rest. I just knew I had to keep driving forward. As if this weren't enough, I added a self-imposed pressure to perform, a well-defined fear of failure or being less than others, residual guilt and shame, and imposter syndrome; now, I would add being directly responsible for the lives of others. Was I good enough for them?

Chapter 7

Uncle Jimmy, the Bear, and the Devil

My great uncle, Uncle Jimmy, was a WWII veteran who served in the Navy aboard the USS Ranger. In 1951, he became a deputy sheriff with the same office I would later work for. He retired as a captain from the office after 33 years of service. Uncle Jimmy was quiet for the most part, but when he spoke, there was much bass in his voice. As a child, I remember him as ten feet tall and bulletproof, with a presence that indicated he was in control of every situation and every room he entered. He looked like a meaner Gunny Highway, tall and lean, with a graying flat top.

After the sheriff's office hired me, I would see Uncle Jimmy at various family functions. With a serious demeanor but a constant jokester, Uncle Jimmy, then in his late 70s, showed all the signs and symptoms one could expect from aging. Each time I saw Uncle Jimmy, at some point when we were alone, he would speak to me about the office and ask how I was getting along. He never shared his experiences with me.

There was something different about Uncle Jimmy during these conversations that I didn't quite understand then.

Softened by age and usually smiling, Uncle Jimmy seemed very serious during these interactions and always asked the same two questions. Have you met the bear? Have you met the devil?

Having a clue but not a complete understanding of what he was asking, I would answer each question with a question: Who is the bear, and who is the devil? His response was always the same: "You will know when you meet them." Then, as if the conversation had never happened, his attention would return to the family function.

Uncle Jimmy passed away in April 2005 without my answering his questions or him imparting the answers. By this point, I had experienced quite a bit and had my share of *excitement*, as well as *little t and big T* trauma, but I still could not answer the question. As you read this, I assume you have reasoned your way to the answers to Uncle Jimmy's questions and are probably assigning your experiences, incidents, and events to each category.

If you spend long enough in this profession, you will reach a point where you have to meet one or the other, and it becomes immediately apparent why Uncle Jimmy asked these questions. I learned that the *bear* is the person your dad always warned you about. The one person out there that is bigger and meaner than you and looking to kick your ass. I have met my fair share of people intent on doing me harm over a 25-year career. Despite my imposing presence and assured demeanor, there were times when I could not reason with them. On those occasions, a mix of my training and brute force always carried me through.

Throughout my career, I was never pushed, pulled, punched, or kicked in a fight or while taking someone into custody. I was always quick to act rather than to react as dangerous situations presented themselves. I was comfortable with violence and never took a suspect's aggression or actions as personal. Though I have experienced twisted ankles and boxer fractures, which have been my own doing, I cannot attest that I can take a punch. I mean a real punch delivered by someone with the intent to injure or kill me. Though many have tried, one has yet to land.

You may not encounter the *Bear,* but in our professions, we will inevitably be faced with evil, with horrible events that shock the senses and sear themselves into the fabric of our being. This brings us to the question of the *devil.* The *devil* is unmistakable. There is evil, and then there is the *devil.* A meeting with the devil overshadows all others; it sends the feeling of icy fingers down your spine, and you immediately know that you have met them. The *devil* looks through you, like staring into a doll's eyes, vacant of expression. The *devil* is evil in its purest form, whose acts are unfathomable by any human measure. The *devil* feeds on whatever bit of good is left within you and takes a piece of your soul with it.

Uncle Jimmy's questions, once enigmatic, became profound lessons in the realities of law enforcement. They spoke to the dual nature of our profession: confronting physical threats with courage and skill and facing moral and existential challenges that test the limits of one's spirit. Reflecting on these encounters, I understand now why Uncle Jimmy posed those questions—guiding me to recognize and navigate the extremes of human experience, both in the streets and within myself.

The Things We Don't Talk About

During a twenty-five-year career in the country's twelfth-largest law enforcement agency, you can imagine the volume of calls we handled as an organization. To add scope, in my last full year, 2022, we reached over 1,000,000 CAD (Computer-Aided Dispatch) calls, and by mid-2023, we were on pace to crush that number. The patrol district I was assigned to most of my patrol career was one of the most densely populated in the county. The district covered over 100 square miles of land, and the deputies assigned answered, on average, 200,000 CAD calls annually. I spent seventeen years in this district and two in another, rougher part of the county.

In that span of time, I have seen countless deaths by just about any conceivable means, method, mechanism, and state of decomposition. I remember the first and last, the ones I couldn't save, and some that just could not be explained. I have encountered men who tested me physically and the *devil* who peeled away parts of my soul. I remember the calls, the sounds, the smells of charred flesh, and scenes so bloody that you could taste it like a penny in your mouth. I remember the faces but only a few of the names. Some of the names I never bothered to ask. I lived where I worked and had an experience in just about every corner of the north part of the county. There was no escape, and I took no time to reset.

These experiences, though profound, were often left unspoken. Amid the job's demands, there was little room for openly processing the emotional toll of such events. The culture of stoicism prevailed, with incidents often reduced to brief discussions or overlooked entirely once the immediate tasks were completed.

My decision to document these events in writing later in life allowed me to explore their significance more deeply. It became apparent that these were not just isolated tragedies but part of a broader narrative of human suffering and resilience that law enforcement officers witness daily.

These scenes represent just a fraction of law enforcement's

profound and often unspoken realities. They underscore the importance of reflection, both for personal growth and to honor the lives and stories that shaped my career. Each encounter, whether with tragedy or resilience, left an indelible mark on my journey—a journey defined by the things we often don't talk about but carry with us nonetheless.

Chapter 8

Scene 1, Death From Below

The date was September 28, 1998, and I was in the early days of phase three of field training and assigned to the night shift. In the middle of the shift, just after midnight, we were dispatched to the hospital to investigate an allegation of potential child neglect or abuse. The comments in the call informed us that a two-year-old boy had arrived at the emergency room by ambulance. Both parents were present and waiting in the reception area. The call notes advised that the boy was possibly reacting to yellow jacket stings. Again, this is midnight, and yellow jackets are not nocturnal. It is safe to say this was delayed.

My field training officer (FTO) and I arrived at the hospital and went straight to the pediatric emergency room. We were hustled into the treatment room, where a doctor and nurses were working to revive the child. The child was in a diaper, and I noticed he was covered in purple welts. This was not an allergic reaction to *a* yellow jacket sting but a reaction to hundreds of yellow jacket stings. Standing at the bedside, the doctor pronounced the child dead one hour after he arrived.

The doctor explained the situation to us before informing the parents that their son was dead. We learned that the child and his parents were visiting from the other coast, and the child was in the backyard around 5 p.m. when he walked into a yellow jacket nest. Yellow jackets build nests underground, are very aggressive if their colony is disturbed, and can deliver multiple stings, unlike bees. The child only wore shorts and shoes when he fell into the nest. He was stung everywhere not covered by clothing.

The parents told the doctor that they thought the child would be okay after they bathed him and let him watch television. Furthermore, the parents said the child acted normally, and they put him to bed later in the evening. It was not until they found him unresponsive just before midnight that they called EMS, nearly seven hours after their son had walked into a yellow jacket nest!

This was my first time seeing a dead child. His tiny, lifeless body was covered in purple welts; he just lay there, expressionless. We took photos, and I started my report while we waited for the medical examiner to arrive. Later, the medical examiner arrived at the hospital with a crime scene technician, and they began taking pictures of the body. The medical examiner moved the child around to locate more stings on the child's back. She found yellow jacket stingers on the back of the child's head under his hairline. It was remarkable, but a yellow jacket had stung him multiple times on the forehead, creating an arc pattern. In total, the child had been stung 432 times. I could not imagine the pain that the baby endured.

My field training officer met with the parents when the detectives arrived. The detectives introduced themselves and started their interview. The parents provided the same story to the detectives as they did to the medical staff. The detectives asked why they did not seek medical attention earlier; they replied that their religion prevents them from seeking medical assistance and reporting births or deaths. So, no doctors or medicine? It was at this point that I excused myself from the interview. I was on the verge of rage, not only in response to the parents' negligence but for their reason why they did not seek medical attention. I get it; they're devout followers of their religion with no doctors and no medicine. What I did not get was that if doctors were *sorcerers* and their medicine potions, someone should be able to explain why mom had Caladryl lotion on her few yellow jacket stings and was wearing prescription eyeglasses and their child got nothing.

I went back into the pediatric ER where the child was located. I sat at the bedside, writing my report, seething about the entire event until the medical examiner removed the child. My field training officer and I never spoke of the incident again. Two days later, an article was published in the Tampa Tribune, and I cut it out and added it to the now-growing trauma collection. I still have the article in an ammo can in the closet on the shelf, so shoving trauma into little boxes was figurative and literal.

I was never subpoenaed for the trial, and both parents were acquitted of all charges in August 2000. I wondered if my report was not as complete as it could have been or if there was any other shortfall. I do know that my reports were never lacking from that day forward. Would that little boy have survived with early intervention? I know he would be about 27 years old today if he had.

I was more focused on why they did not seek medical attention earlier, and I was numb while writing a report seated next to a dead child. I was more disappointed that I could not rationalize a reason for this tragedy. I never discussed my reaction to this call with anyone.

Chapter 9

Scene 2, I Couldn't Save Them August-September 1998

Note: *There is nothing peaceful or graceful about CPR. It's quick, stressful, and violent.*

Phases one and two of field training presented abundant opportunities to acquaint myself with death. I responded to a total of seven death investigations, two of which occurred on the same night. Throughout this period, I performed CPR on three occasions, and unfortunately, all three individuals passed away right before my eyes, lying on the floor.

The first of that month's seven deaths sticks with me and has caused the most introspection. We were dispatched to a *person down* call around the corner from where we were. Upon arrival, an older man guided us into the living room. He explained that his wife was sitting in her chair eating the dinner he had prepared when she suddenly stopped responding. We swiftly assessed the situation and moved the lady to the floor to begin CPR. We didn't have Ambu bags then, so we used small one-way valve masks. After checking for vitals and ensuring an open airway, we initiated compressions. My field training officer, or FTO, took charge of the compressions while I focused on maintaining the airway and breathing.

After about three rounds of compressions and breaths, the lady vomited into my mask, and then she was gone. Fire Rescue arrived at the scene, ran a tape, and confirmed no cardiac rhythm. She had passed away right before my eyes as I was trying to get an airway again. Her husband of sixty years was standing by my side. He watched the entire episode unfold on the living room floor in a house that undoubtedly hosted many Thanksgiving and Christmas dinners full of family members and memories. This would have been an occasion that marked a time in someone's life.

I couldn't help but wonder if the compressions were too deep or not deep enough or if I failed to get a good airway. Perhaps it was simply her time to go. Nonetheless, she and I were face to face as her life slipped away. Her family started arriving as we began our documentation process and assisted in removing the body. This experience made me contemplate death on a more personal level. How could I not? Her husband was there the whole time, never leaving her side. I wished I could have brought her back, even for a moment, so she could see him there, knowing he was by her side.

Until this call, I never really had a problem with death theoretically because I knew it was an inevitable part of life. I thought I understood it, but I never considered its finality until I began my career as a law enforcement officer and, specifically, during this call—the close and personal encounter with Death in the room, the Reaper.

Since then, I have given breaths and compressions, held hands, or tried to stop the bleeding as people slip from this life. Amidst the chaos before Death's arrival, I remained professional and unwavering, capable of handling any scene, regardless of its complexity. Master of my shit! However, I could feel the Reaper in the room, pushing past us as he took them. In those instances, if only for an instant, I needed to reset. I never told anyone about this; who was there to tell anyway? This remained my secret, hidden from view in my shadow.

Chapter 10

Scene 3, Date Day and the Wandering Eye

In the early winter of 1998, Michelle and I were in Clearwater, Florida, for a lunch date. I had already completed field training and had been cut loose on my own for several weeks. After lunch, we walked to the parking lot. As we approached her car, there was a crash in the intersection in front of the Clearwater Mall, just on the other side of the small hedge row from where we had been standing. A smaller sedan appeared to have driven from the inside through traffic lane against the light and across three lanes of traffic when it was struck in the intersection.

The car came to rest, and I saw two silhouettes in the front seat. The passenger compartment was full of aerosolized white powder and the pungent smell of deployed airbags. I told Michelle to call 911 and ran toward the car to check on the passengers. As luck would have it, an FDNY firefighter on vacation was in traffic and came to assist. I was already checking on both passengers, and he was under the hood, disconnecting the battery.

There were two elderly occupants, a man and his wife.

They appeared to be in their late 70s or early 80s. The woman was in the passenger seat and had been beaten to shit by the passenger side airbag. I initially thought she went into the windshield based on the trauma to her face, but the spider webbing on the windshield came from the airbag deployment. She was dazed but breathing, as indicated by her screams. I wanted to stabilize her but looked at the driver, who was in much worse shape.

From personal experience, an airbag hit me in the chest, and I could not raise my arms above my head for a week; I was young and in shape. The frail older man took the blast straight to the face. I looked at him and had to pause and focus. The man was facing straight ahead through the now smashed windshield but was also staring at me. The impact of the airbag crushed his orbital bone, and his right eye had avulsed and was resting on his cheek.

Well, that seems simple enough unless you are unprepared for what comes next. That was when it became apparent that eyes move in concert with one another, and if one is housed properly, it moves side to side within the socket. All of that is fine if both eyes are inside the socket. But, if one eye is on a fucking walkabout, laying on a cheek, it jumps around like a fish out of water when its owner starts looking around. Now, there was no time to taste my newly acquired Tex-Mex, and I found myself in the backseat of the car, stabilizing the driver's head and neck, trying to convince a man in shock to stare at the dashboard and to stop looking around.

Fire rescue arrived on the scene and decided I was in the best position to keep him stabilized. So, a paramedic placed a cup of some type over the man's eye, put a dressing on his head, and placed a C-collar on him and his wife as they cut away the rear driver's side door. I was relieved by the paramedics as they laid back his seat and slid a backboard underneath him. I met Michelle on the sidewalk and noticed she was white, like my T-shirt.

I was ready to return to the date, and Michelle and I talked about it after we left. She later said she was impressed with how I responded and hoped they would be okay. I remarked that they were landing a medivac, which was not promising. That was about the extent of the conversation.

In the winter of 2023, I asked Michelle if she remembered this date, specifically her recollections. She said she remembered it vaguely but could recall the injuries, the position of the car in the intersection, and, oddly, the car's color. Dates with me were memorable.

Chapter 11

Scene 4, The Airmen and New Boots-1999

As I wrote earlier, Rich and I sat side-by-side in the reserve deputy academy in February 1998. Rich was hired full-time in November 1998, and we went together like peas and carrots (I hope you read that in Forrest Gump's voice). When we were cut loose from the academy and our FTO, we were assigned as zone partners, and we, like most rookies, were active.

We were the scourge of Town and Country, an area in our district's southern part. Rich and I went everywhere together; he was even at my wedding. Rich was, and still is to this day, a great friend and one of the best cops I have ever met. There were no airs; what you saw was what you got, and God help you if you asked for his opinion on something. Twenty-five years after we sat together in class, I finished my career with Rich by my side.

Rich and I have plenty of *no shit there I was* stories with each other. We solved armed robberies and shootings, had car and foot chases, and pulled more dope than anyone else.

Although we were close, we went on a call that we never

spoke about until the day I retired—twenty-four years had passed since the incident. Rich and I would patrol the zone, following each other at a distance but close enough to get to a traffic stop and assist if needed.

One night, Rich turned northbound on Sheldon Road from Hillsborough Avenue. I was about a half mile behind. Then, the radio came to life. Rich came up on the radio and advised that a crash had happened in front of him; one vehicle was on its roof, and the occupants were trapped.

I arrived on the scene just as Rich got on his belly and began crawling into the overturned car. A lot of smoke was coming from the engine compartment, which was never a good sign. I squatted next to Rich and looked into the car. Three bodies were mangled and trapped inside. The front seat occupants were dead, which was evident due to their position, and the passenger's head was oblong and split in half long ways. Rich then started talking to the person in the back seat. He was trapped, in pain, and frantic. Rich could not move him or get into the car any further to free him. Rich held his hand and continued to talk to him. The kid spat out blood and teeth with every word.

The driver of the other vehicle had minor injuries as a result of the crash and was being assisted by deputies arriving on the scene. Deputies began shutting down the roadway and waiting for Fire Rescue to arrive. Their station was around the corner, but it felt like it took hours for them to get there. Fire Rescue arrived, and at this point, the smoke in the engine compartment was now a visible fire. Again, this is a bad sign. Cars and single-wide trailers burn hot and fast.

I told Rich about the fire, and Rich refused to leave the trapped backseat passenger, and the passenger would not let him leave. So, he stayed on his belly halfway inside the car. Fire

Rescue attacked the fire and began placing cribbing on the back of the car so they could stabilize and start cutting people out. These firefighters were fucking fast. What Rich and I did not know and what Rich discovered first was that the collision had all but disintegrated the car's firewall. There was nothing between Rich and the fire except the large volume of water entering the passenger compartment, which caused everything to wash out of the broken windows and into the grass. Luckily, the cribbing in the back of the car tilted it just forward enough to force the water out of the front windows and not into the back seat area where Rich and the survivor were.

Rich stayed in the car, still holding the passenger's hand. I backed up as quickly as I could to avoid the gore and CDs now flowing from the vehicle. As I backed up, my boot slipped on something. I pointed my flashlight to my feet and saw the front seat passenger's brain, which was fully intact, stem and all. I do not know why and have not unraveled this mystery, but I thought then that this was my first night in brand-new boots; I just got the shine right and had not even broken them in. They were later donated to the medical examiner as a biohazard, and I had to drive home in socks.

Everyone was cut out of the car, starting with the patient that Rich was with. Rich never left him alone. He laid on his belly in the car and held the boy's hand the entire time. The firefighters covered him and carefully cut around him to extricate the patient.

However, as the patient was removed, an even more shocking discovery was made – a fourth person in the car. By the end of this call, we would learn that the backseat passengers were brothers. When the car flipped and came to rest on its roof, the patient ended up on top of his brother, completely concealing him from view.

The situation took a devastating turn as we learned more details. The fourth passenger's fingernails were all but pulled off his fingertips. The mystery surrounding this phenomenon was solved when they found claw marks and deep scratches on the survivor's back. It turned out that his brother had survived the initial crash but tragically suffocated to death as he desperately clawed at his brother's back, struggling to get air. Trapped, unable to move, and unable to communicate, upside down in a smoke-filled car, our patient laid atop his brother and smothered him to death.

We remained silent on the scene for the rest of the night, processing what we had seen. As far as resilience and mental health are concerned, we were not aware of any mechanism or protocol for addressing mental health issues at the time, and even if such resources were available, we would not have utilized them. Neither Rich nor I discussed our perspectives on that call until my last day of duty. It was only then that we finally opened up about it. However, the conversation was superficial at best. We were not ready to open the box.

Several weeks after I retired, Rich's mom passed. I have known him for more than 25 years, and though we are not brothers, I feel as close to him as any other, and I know his heart. He is a very private person, and I was not aware that his mother had passed. Although he had been on my mind for over a week, I did not reach out to find out how he and his family were doing. When I did, I learned his mother had passed.

Moving past the level of shit friend that I am, I heard something in his voice in our conversation that I had never heard before. The following day, I saw him at the district and brought him his favorite lunch: a Costco hot dog. Rich and I had the most meaningful and open conversation we ever had together. It occurred to me that despite how close he and I had been for so many years, we never discussed any of the traumatic calls we ran together. I wonder if it would have made a difference.

This thought raises more questions than answers. Was our silence a conscious choice out of fear, stigma, or an inability for us, as men, to be vulnerable in front of each other? Was this the culture of the veteran and responder communities then, and to a large degree still, to not be vulnerable in fear that it would be seen as a weakness? Most importantly, what does this say about us as friends?

Chapter 12

Scene 5, The Dead Cat and Moral Injury

On a Friday night in the summer of 2000, I was dispatched to a welfare check with the Department of Children and Family Services (DCFS) following an anonymous complaint. The report suggested that children were living in deplorable conditions, neglected, and under the care of a mother struggling with drug addiction. This was a common practice, and we routinely responded with DCFS when there was a criminal allegation or the possibility of removing children from the home and placing them into protective custody.

The residence was a single-wide trailer offset from the road on a piece of property behind a ranch-style home. The home belonged to the children's grandfather, and the residents of the trailer were, of course, his grandchildren, son, and daughter-in-law.

I met with the person from child services at the base of the driveway leading to the trailer. She informed me that the complaint was anonymous and alleged the children were being cared for by their mother, who was an addict, and their father was rarely home as he worked long hours. Furthermore, the grandfather who lived on the property was no help, and the children, quite frankly, ran loose most days.

Walking down the dirt driveway, I saw two young children sitting in the path, petting a cat lying in the dirt between them. The cat was surprisingly relaxed, considering neither child was particularly gentle. The mother met us in the driveway just before we reached the children. We introduced ourselves and asked if we could speak with her inside her residence. I noticed the children were dirt-covered and likely had not bathed in days. We walked toward the house, and I looked at the cat, still lying in the path, as we passed by. The cat's eyes were wide open and opaque. The cat was dead, at least for the day, and the kids played with it as if it were all *nimbly pimbly* (meow). Oh, it does not end here.

There were garbage bags full of raw garbage stacked like so many cords of split wood. They were stacked against the wall and reached from the ground to the carport's roof. This was not only unsanitary but also lazy. The property was a quarter-mile walk to the dump.

We were invited in, and the inside was just as disgusting as the outside, but with carpet—spoiled food on plates and not one square foot of clean space inside the entire trailer. Not soon after we walked inside, I recommended that DCF remove all children and place them into protective custody. She agreed and went outside to call her supervisors and start the removal process. I contacted my supervisor and let her know the possible outcome.

A removal seemed to be the obvious move in this event because the mother had an addiction, was incapable or disinterested in caring for the children, the conditions were deplorable, and the father was nowhere to be found. The DCF investigator returned to speak with the mother while I spoke with my supervisor.

While I was gone, she found out the mother had planned to leave for Alabama the next day with her children so her mother could care for them while she was at an in-patient treatment facility in Alabama. DCF decided to document the case and forward it to their counterparts in Alabama for a follow-up.

I passionately opposed the plan of forwarding the case to DCFS counterparts in Alabama and was very vocal about my concerns. Allowing someone to remove children who I felt were being neglected to leave our jurisdiction and take them to a jurisdiction that was not familiar with what we experienced at the scene was a mistake. I voiced my concerns to my supervisor and was told that DCF had jurisdiction over the case and that we would abide by their recommendation. I stood in the driveway, watching the mother and her children drive away.

I assumed that inpatient drug rehabilitation programs lasted roughly a month and that we would be dispatched to DCF when they did a follow-up. However, there was no digital report database, and accessing DCF files was unheard of, so I waited to be dispatched to a follow-up call with DCF.

Unfortunately, the follow-up would come three weeks after our initial call, but in the form of a child drowning. As fate would have it, the mother never went to rehab in Alabama and returned home with the children days after they left.

The children were left in the grandfather's care at his house on the property. He was less than capable of caring for children, if not wholly negligent, and was not keeping track of the children. The two older children were playing inside, and the toddler was found face down in the bottom of the backyard pool. The child was transported to All Children's Hospital, and

I sat at the hospital all night with detectives and the parents until the child was removed from life support.

I understand that the primary goal is to protect children and keep the family intact if at all possible. But, this was one call that I could not reason through. Being right or wrong at this point did not matter.

It would take several years before I could pass by that corner the trailer sat on without thinking about that call. Years later, the corner lot was bulldozed and replaced with a Costco.

Chapter 13

Scene 6, Keep Your Finger Off the Trigger

I was assigned to the training division, and my duties included coordinating an academy class. In December 2006, my class went to the range. I visited them as other instructors were running the course of instruction that day. Not long after I arrived, the students were doing individual shooting drills. This drill required one person and two instructors, as they would be moving on the line and engaging discretionary targets.

Punch it out, charge, and holster your loaded weapon were the commands given to the recruits. The instructor would pause to allow the recruits to adjust themselves; then, the instructor would begin the set of drills by saying *up*. Each drill followed this sequence, but one. The command set of *punch it out, charge, and holster your loaded weapon* was given and was followed by the unmistakable sound of a pistol firing. My back was turned when the discharge occurred, and by the time I turned and my eyes focused, I saw my recruit. He was now on the ground writhing in pain after sending a .40 caliber FMJ (full metal jacket) round through his upper thigh, shattering his femur, and coming to rest in the inner lower leg just above the ankle. The round was still inside, just under the skin. When he holstered the pistol, the recruit had his finger inside the trigger guard. The instructors, who were seasoned professionals, began treating the recruit as I ran to them with my IFAK (Individual First Aid Kit). We controlled the bleeding and kept him stable for the thirty-minute response from Fire/Rescue as the range was in the middle of nowhere.

The wounded recruit was retired from the military, a great leader, fit, and tough as nails. He lay on the ground, gritting his teeth and shaking his head in disbelief at what he had just done. The class watched the entire event in real-time, from when it occurred to when the recruit was transported to the hospital. Later that night, my recruit would undergo an hours-long surgery to repair the bones and the damage done by the round.

The next day, with titanium rods for a femur, surrounded by shredded muscle, this man had already been walking from his room to the nurses' station. He wanted to recover and get back to his class. I met him the night after his surgery; he sat in bed and addressed me as sir. I shook his hand and told him I cut his pants off, and we held hands in the dirt for thirty minutes; we were well past him addressing me as sir. He recovered and was later hired by a municipal agency within the county. The last word I heard was that he was a supervisor and member of the SWAT team at a local municipal agency. There was no quit in him.

My missed opportunity here was that I never addressed this with the class. They saw their friend, the class leader, suffer what would have been, for a lesser person, a career-ending injury. I thanked the two instructors, who were on top of their game, but we never spoke about its impact on either of us. I also never talked about the impact of seeing one of my troops wounded on the ground. These things never occurred to me at that moment. It is in the quiet of not doing that you unravel these events.

Chapter 14

Scene 7, We Went to Work
August 8, 2007

I had multiple one-liners ready for just about any occasion. During my time in the Training Division, one in particular was *Go to Work!*

In late July 2007, I transferred out of the Training Division and returned to my district. I was assigned a recruit named Mark C. He was a member of the academy class I coordinated, and I knew what he could do because I had seen him daily for eight months. Our time together was an excellent opportunity to evaluate and validate my training methods, and there was no shortage of surprises.

It was the week of August 6, 2007. Summer in Central Florida was in full swing, and Mark was early in phase two of his training. On August 8, we worked the afternoon shift from 1300 to 0100 hours. Mark came to work, pleased with himself, and handed me a DVD of the film 300. He told me to take it home and watch it before I returned to work the next day. He and other class members had been urging me to watch it for several weeks.

I took the DVD and threw it in the trunk of my patrol car.

Doug White

We always took my car. Why? Because I'm driving, and a recruit is not going to wreck my car. Also, and more importantly, I had my AR, hundreds of 5.56 rounds, and three spare Glock magazines stuffed with .40 caliber duty ammo in the door panels of the driver and passenger side of the vehicle. Rule number one in a gunfight is not to run out of bullets, and we wouldn't. I also had breaching charges, counter-charges, explosives, heavy armor, a helmet, and an entry shield that I liberated from the SWAT team to round out my traveling kit.

But today, we took Mark's car because I was tired of him whining about when he could stop to pee or buy another Monster. So, off we went. Mark went to 7-11, got his Monster, and then to the next stop.

There were a few rules when I was in the car; the primary was don't shit yourself in the car, and before any enforcement action–Doug gets coffee. I was unbendable on this one.

Mark drove into the drive-thru of a free-standing building where they sold coffee from a Seattle-based company. The drive-through was not a habit, but it was hot outside, and I just got situated on the passenger side of the Crown Vic. Like many recruits, Mark knew my drink order and ordered for me. While waiting in line, a call was voiced for a welfare check/contact message in a neighborhood behind the district.

The call comments told us that the caller was worried about their son and had not heard from him, so he wanted us to check on him. We were not in the area but had just gotten a stack of Baker Act paperwork, and I saw this as a training opportunity. I told him we would take the training call and put us on the call when we got out of the drive-through. As fate would have it, a motor unit was on her way home and would pass by the location in just a few minutes. Mark put us on the call, and we retrieved my drink.

Approximately 45 minutes into our shift and in traffic working our way to the call, the motor unit got on the radio and advised us that she had arrived on the scene. For some reason, and I cannot explain it to this day, I told Mark to step on the accelerator if she returned to the radio, and her voice was *different*. Seconds later, she keyed up.

"*He's signal o*," (armed), she said.

That was Mark's cue to step on it. In retrospect, her tone was remarkably calm for someone greeted by a .357 revolver to her face.

I was not paying attention to Mark driving, although some scrapes were in the median. I brought up the map and noted we would drive by the district office—the perfect time to get my car and *go to work*.

More updates were coming in, and we were the closest. I thought, "Shit! There's no time to stop!" We passed the district and turned into the subdivision. Checking the map, I told Mark there was no vantage point or cover that would allow us to see the side of the house we needed to cover. Our only option was to park adjacent to the house on the street and use the car for cover. This was imperfect.

Update: the motor unit advised it was a single male who, when he answered the door, had a large caliber revolver behind his back. He told her to leave or *bad things* would happen. She asked what he meant, and he put the gun in her face and said *someone would die*. He let her go. She retreated to the front of the driveway and took cover behind her vehicle. Luckily, she was in her car and not on the motorcycle.

The scene: a single-level block stucco structure on the corner of the main street and a cul-de-sac. The main door to the house was on the side of the house, facing the street. A six-foot tall, dog-eared wood privacy fence surrounded the backyard, mainly concealing the roofed back patio and the shed. As it was past noon, we could see movement and silhouettes between the fence slats, and the backyard was backlit from our vantage point.

We announced our arrival and position and switched all traffic to a tactical channel to free the main channel. As with all hot calls, everyone wants to get in on the action. We held the station, but everyone decided to voice their en route status rather than drive and get there. In short, there is no radio for Doug, Mark, and the motor unit. I told Mark to take the front, giving him the engine block, and took the trunk, hoping the full-size spare and all of his unnecessary shit would stop a round should one find its way to me.

A moment after we arrived, we were joined by another deputy, who was also on his way home. We will call him Al for anonymity. Al drove in from the north, whereas we approached from the south. He queued off our location, stopped on the north end of the privacy fence, and exited his car about thirty feet from the front of our car. Mark was between us, and I could not fully see Al other than gross movements from my peripheral.

Now, Al was an old-school deputy; they kept their concealable armor in the trunk and would retrieve it if needed. Well, the need presented itself. Al went to his trunk and put on his vest. He returned to the driver's side door, which he had left open. Standing by the door, Al got on the radio and said he heard the screen porch door open. Just then, all hell broke loose!

With one hand on his radio and one on the A pillar of his driver-side door, Al stood fully exposed fifteen feet from the fence, almost perfectly aligned with the porch door. One blast in the air, *BOOM!* Then, as Al pushed the car door shut, the largest Mossberg 590 shotgun presented itself over the top of the fence, wielded by our suspect, hell-bent on killing one or all of us.

The second shot was well-aimed, and BOOM, a slug went through the windshield of Al's car. A 12-gauge slug entered Al's car and out through the driver's side door window as Al was closing it. The round shattered the glass, sending Al straight back onto the ground. Al was down!

The suspect took another shot at Al, and I could see his silhouette through the slats on the fence. I saw a white tank top, a T-shirt, and a shotgun. I was at a 45-degree angle and about forty-five feet from the suspect. I leaned out from the back of the car, sight picture, sight alignment, breath and trigger control, squeeze, and recoil. Now aware of our intent to fight back, the suspect started moving down the fence toward us and away from Al. Mark said he's moving to us. Just then, the shotgun emerges once more. Mark takes cover; BOOM! Mark is back up and ready to respond. Mark said he was moving to the gate. By this time, I was focused on the gate.

Intent on the gate, I saw a hand reach around the side of the gate from behind. The gate swung open, and the suspect presented himself. Here we go. Now, about forty feet away, at a slight angle, I am facing a person with a white t-shirt leveling a shotgun at me. *Recoil, recoil!* BOOM! A controlled pair performed as I had done thousands of times in training. The suspect answered my shots in perfect synchronicity as he fired and retreated from view.

Mark and I knew he was standing in the backyard, at the corner of the fence, hidden from view and reloading. We knew we could not let him make it to the street. Knowing our backstop was a block house, we were relatively sure he was in the corner. We both went to work emptying our magazines into the corner of the fence. I recall taking cover to reload. I had counted my rounds and had one left in the breach. Hundreds of hours of counting rounds in training paid off. Now, six feet away, Mark, a mirror image, locked eyes with me, and we were back up. Mark said he could see him on the ground. He had fallen back and now had just enough light to make out the silhouette.

Al was down!

I shouted, "Get to Al; he's down!"

I covered the fence line as Mark did a remarkable thing. This crazy bastard did precisely what he was told. Without hesitation, he left cover, pistol in hand, and I saw him moving away from me in my peripheral. He grabbed Al, dragged him to the front of his car, and leaned him against the front tire. He checked him for holes, finding none; he placed Al's radio in one hand and his pistol in the other. Then, Mark came back to me. He was panting after covering roughly 60 feet of fully exposed real estate. Knowing Al was sans holes, I told him to return to Al; he needs you there. I did not finish my sentence, and this silly bastard left cover and went to Al: ninety feet now, the distance between home plate and first base. Balls out exposed. Additional deputies began to arrive, and now Al had company. Mark decided to come back one more time to keep me company. 120 feet!

I updated the dispatcher that the subject was down, and we were ten-four, and we heard other deputies were en route. The *shotgun opera* could be heard clearly from the district office, and everyone came to the rescue. We now have 11th-hour heroes staging around the corner while Mark, the initial unit, Al, and deputies just joined Al sitting or standing on asphalt. In August-in Florida, in the heat of the day. I don't have the patience for this. Aviation arrived on the scene but could not get an angle due to the canopy, and they did not want to get over the suspect in the event he could still shoot.

So, SWAT was called. SWAT is the best in the business, but the team still has a potential 30-minute window while we were baking in polyester pants and armor—it was time to devise a plan. I looked at Mark and told him to get in the car, stay low, put the car in drive, and break the fence while I walked astride as I used the car for cover. Check! Mark was all in and moving to the door when the sergeant, knowing me well enough, got on the radio and said, "Doug White, stay put." Well, damn.

The staging deputies and detectives decided they would make the entry into the backyard and check the suspect. These 11th-hour heroes looked ridiculous as they approached. About ten deputies and detectives were in a wedge, shotguns in the front and the others, pistols in hand, formed at the end of the block. They tactically approached as I watched them walk heel-toe from a block away. They stealthily approached and made entry. The suspect was dead; a single gunshot wound entered his upper left chest, piercing the lung, severing the aorta, and stopping between the skin and right shoulder blade.

Detectives and supervisors arrived, followed closely by the crime scene. There had been a shooting, and there was a process to ensure that the conditions were justifiable and policy was met. This orchestrated chaos was necessary and prevented me from returning to work. So, there we were. No one had spoken to us. Mark and I were standing side by side in the street, watching the investigation unfold.

Now, there is a certain way that I stand, a posture I take when I am aggravated: feet shoulder-width apart, hands on my hips, head lowered, but sure to make eye contact- staring through the object of my disdain. If we have worked together, at one point in time, you have seen the stance or at least the piercing stare.

There we were, standing in the street. I looked down and noticed I had two shadows. How was this possible? I looked at Mark, and be damned if he wasn't in the same stance. I guess months with me were just long enough to imprint on the *I'm not pleased look*.

The chief deputy, as did a couple of colonels, showed up on the scene. Other than my sergeant, they were the first to address me. Standing at the back of Mark's car, I met the chief deputy and colonel and told them what happened. I introduced them to Mark and informed them that Mark was today's hero. I explained how he ran to Al across open real estate to check on him while the scene was still active. To this very day, I believe Mark was the hero on that call. We were right where we were supposed to be when we were supposed to be there.

Al's car was towed away when he was transported by Fire/Rescue for observation. He bashed his head pretty good and was out cold. Looking at Al's car, we saw the first round fired, the one that went through the windshield and out the driver-side window, shearing off the handcuff chains from the handcuffs hanging from his spotlight handle. Man, that was close. The next round on Al was in the middle of the hood, just short of where he was on the ground. That was when I fired my first round. Detectives still do not understand how my first round missed the suspect.

Looking at Mark's car from the suspect's vantage point, there was a 12-gauge slug-sized hole in the green construction screen surrounding a dirt lot on our side of Mark's car. This hole was about eighteen inches above the hood and in a direct line with the center of the front tire. Mark would have taken that round to the face if he had not moved to cover. We walked to the trunk of Mark's car, and there was a 12-gauge slug-sized hole in the rear driver-side quarter panel, directly adjacent to where I was when I fired the controlled pair. The suspect fired his last round, which skipped off the asphalt short of the car, and the slug ricocheted into the quarter panel. Any slower in our response, and I would have caught that round with my torso.

Detectives would conclude that the suspect was already on the ground when Mark and I unleashed our salvo into the corner of the fence. That was a good thing; he would have a whole lot of bullets had he been on his feet. Based on the wound, he was dead before he hit the ground. I never saw the body after the incident. I had closure. He tried to kill us, and he did not. There, closure. I never read the coroner's report. As far as I know, that round could have been mine, just as likely as Mark's. We both made the conscious decision to fire and stop the threat, and together, we shouldered the weight of being forced to take his life.

We spent the rest of the afternoon and evening in the district, answering questions and taking oaths. At about 2100 hours, we were driven home.

Michelle was at home with both kids, two years old and six months old. I called her earlier, after the incident, and told her there was an issue and that we were all okay. This was a good phone call, considering my wife was just about to drive past the street on her way home from her mom's house. We had an agreement when we began dating seriously. If I call you, everything is okay, and I will be home when I can. If someone else calls or knocks, get in the fucking car, it's bad. I do not know that Michelle and I ever spoke about this incident from an "are you okay" perspective. If so, I inevitably shut it down.

I was at home, and the sheriff called me later that night. He was a great man who wanted to check in on me, which meant a lot. I slept like a baby that night. I suspect it was an effect of the adrenaline dump and relief that all of my training and my efforts with Mark's class and their ability to learn and perform were enough to get us all home.

The following day, I watched 300 for the first time. It was a great movie. However, finishing the movie 45 minutes before you go to the psyche to hear about what he thinks you should be experiencing after a deadly force encounter was, in retrospect, a terrible idea. I just smiled and envisioned myself kicking him into a bottomless pit.

Later that day, Al called me. He spent the night in the hospital and had a nasty bump on the back of his head. I should note that this was Al's fifth involvement in a deadly force encounter in as many years. Nevertheless, he was there. I had known Al for a while, and although we had not worked together, he was aware of my reputation.

I did not have an issue with the incident or how we performed. We went home. As far as I was concerned, there was no sliding scale of success; you either go home or you don't. This changed after Al called me. Again, this was his fifth and his closest to that point.

Al confided in me that he had arrived and saw Mark and me behind the car. So, he went to his trunk to get his vest. He said he heard the porch door open, and then all hell broke loose. He had his radio in his hand and was shutting the door when the blast from the window shattering pushed him off balance. He said he fell straight back and hit his head on the street. He was out, and he did not know how long. He said he heard a pistol shot, then a shotgun blast from in front of his vehicle. I told him this was when the suspect was walking down the fence line and fired a round on Mark.

He broke down. He said he was coming to when he heard the shot from in front of his vehicle. He said he thought the suspect had gotten out of the backyard. Al said he thought the suspect was coming around the front of his car and he was going to die. He said he could not see the suspect but knew he was there and he was about to die. He said he pulled his pistol and fired one round toward the front of his car and lost consciousness again. He said the next thing he remembered was waking and hearing another blast from the front of his car and a lot of pistols.

He told me that he had never met Mark and had no idea who he was, but he looked past Mark and saw me shooting. He then said he laid his head back and thought, *Doug is here, I'm not going to die today.* He then passed out again and woke up when Mark grabbed him and dragged him to his car.

This was the only thing I consciously carried with me after this incident. Al's phone call was the one thing, the one feeling that seared into my mind—the persona. Living up to the story that is built around you is emotionally draining. When someone tells you that they believed they were going to die and fired a round out of desperation, then only after seeing you was assured that they would live. That everything will be okay. It's the heaviest burden I have ever carried. The fear of letting someone down was now tucked in the shadow.

Eleven months later, Al was in another deadly force encounter-a full-on gunfight where another deputy and Al were shot by a suspect in a homicide. This was Al's sixth shooting in as many years. He recovered and retired shortly after his recovery.

Neither Mark nor I spoke about the shooting outside of the interviews. We did not share our perspectives. Although we spoke several times and spent quite a bit of time together during our time off during the investigation, we did not speak about it until after the state's attorney cleared us 21 days later. The extended time was due to another incident, when in the week following our shooting, one of our sergeants was ambushed and murdered.

Mark and I returned to duty, and the first thing we did was drive back to the scene and park in the same spot we were in three weeks earlier. We both shared our perspectives and walked through the entire scene. For three weeks, I believed that if we were in my car and I had my rifle, we would have ended the confrontation after the subject's first shot. Walking through the scene put this thought to rest. Based on my angle that day and the apparent angle of the subject, had I missed with the rifle, the 5.56 round may have traveled into the neighbor's house and not the shed adjacent to the subject, as my pistol round had. The pistol was the right choice, and I never considered the issue again.

Mark and I were good with our actions and the outcome. Ironically, our first call on our first day back was a man with a shotgun threatening his family. I recall no one was keen on going to the call with us.

There was no follow-up by the office or further contact from the contracted psychologist. Then, and to this day, I am emotionally neutral to the personal impact of having a hand in taking a human life. I never gave it another thought. Now, I realize either my capacity for emotion was diminished, if not gone, before this incident, or I was good at compartmentalizing. Either way, it's not healthy.

Chapter 15

Scene 8, The Weekend: The Devil, the Duffel, and the Angel
March 8-10, 2009

It is often said that bad news comes in groups of three. March 6-8, 2009, would mark my career's worst incident streak. A single three-day work weekend, thirty-six hours of trauma between Friday and Sunday, and there was no hiding from it. The first and third events, Friday and Sunday, were so awful that, to this day, I cannot recall what happened on Saturday. The brain is a powerful organ, and I assume that there is a mechanism that shuts down when events become too much to process. My research of this vignette caused me to search for the suspects' names on the Department of Correction website to go back to the offense date and search for the news article from the incident. I have not and will not research the call log from Saturday. I will let this monster lie.

What happened on Friday? A woman passed out in a restaurant bathroom and gave birth to a little girl. The mother was found unresponsive on the floor. The baby was face down in the toilet with the umbilical cord wrapped around her neck. We were literally in the intersection when the call came in, and it would not have made a difference. The father was next door with his young son getting a haircut while the mom waited at the restaurant to have lunch afterward.

Sunday

> *For the intent and purpose of this next vignette, I will refer to the parties as the female suspect (mom), the male suspect (boyfriend), the boy, and the angel (the victim). I will never speak the names of those responsible for this incident because, fuck them. The names I use once are for emphasis and are fictitious.*

On Sunday, March 8, 2009, our shift began at 0600 hours, and my recruit was scheduled to meet me at the district office. This plan had been unchanged since I started training recruits in 1999. I was the most senior trainer in the district, so supervisors would depend on me more often than not to *sort the unsorted* or to handle the more complex issues or recruits. The sergeant or platoon commander calling me early before or during a shift to divert or dispatch me directly was common.

My phone rang at 0530 hours, just as I left my house. The sergeant requested that I pick my recruit up and respond directly to the primary incident scene. She informed me that another day shift unit would respond with detectives to the hospital and relieve the night shift who had arrived with the ambulance. She explained that the night shift was on the scene at an extended stay efficiency motel, where a child had been transported from, and she needed me to go to the scene, relieve the supervisor, and assume the investigation. I volunteered to go to the hospital, and she quickly repeated that I would under no circumstance go to the hospital and that I was needed on the scene to relieve the supervisor. Her tone was unusual, and I thought it was strange since we both knew I was closer to the hospital than I was to the incident scene. Nevertheless, I picked up my recruit and went to the initial scene.

On the way to the scene, we reviewed the initial call and the investigative notes to bring us up to speed. I directed the recruit to his resources and broadly went over our work priorities in general when investigating a crime and the investigative resources available in these cases. Neither he nor I could have anticipated what we would encounter over the next several hours. We arrived on the scene, and I met with the night shift sergeant. He confirmed the information we reviewed in the call notes and explained they wanted me there early before the night shift became too involved to be able to back out. Again, this was not an uncommon practice.

The sergeant then directed me to the small efficiency room, the incident scene. He explained that a female infant was transported to All Children's Hospital by fire rescue, and she was unresponsive. He was not sure of her status or prognosis. He told me a young boy was sitting in the room with another deputy, and the children's mother was speaking with child protective investigators just as we arrived.

I noticed a male, the suspect, sitting on a stool at the end of the hallway with a deputy standing next to him. My attention immediately went to the male suspect on the stool. He was sitting straight up in a stoic, if not indignant or defiant posture. I had not caught his eye, but he caught mine.

I continued to the room and saw a young boy sitting on the bed with a female deputy inside the room. The child appeared cheerful or at least relieved. I greeted the deputy and looked at the little boy. I noticed someone had used a permanent marker and wrote "Dumbass" on his forehead.

The little boy looked at me and said, "*Joey (the suspect) killed Debbie (the angel).*"

I told my recruit to write that down. I assumed the suspect on the stool was *Joey*.

Now that I had a handle on the scene and requested the necessary resources, I called my sergeant at the hospital. I told her everything was well in hand and asked how the patient was doing. There was a pause and then a shaky response. She said she was unsure, which I later discovered was untrue. Nevertheless, I continued with the scene. The detectives arrived, and my recruit took over the crime scene log. I would relieve the deputy, keeping tabs on the male suspect.

I turned my attention back to the male suspect, who was still defiantly perched on his stool. He made eye contact with me just as I started to walk in his direction. As soon as we made eye contact, his defiant posture shrunk, and he stared at the ground. His demeanor changed so rapidly that I asked the deputy what happened. It was a mystery to both of us.

I introduced myself to the male suspect and asked for his identification. I wanted to have the information and a criminal history for the detectives before they arrived. The suspect was difficult to understand, almost whispering. I did not ask for further information, and he offered nothing—just as well, less for me to write.

The child protective investigators, district and CID detectives, and crime scene technicians arrived relatively close to one another. I knew the child at the hospital was either deceased or expected when I noticed CID detectives arriving. After a while, another deputy arrived on the scene, and the detectives requested them to transport the male suspect to the district office for questioning. Child protection took the little boy into protective custody and transported him to the hospital for treatment. Later, when the scene was closed, my recruit and I transported the children's mother to the district for further questioning.

The mother told my recruit and I her life story in the ten-minute drive to the district. She had met the male suspect a couple of months prior online while playing an online game, and they had been living together in the efficiency for a few weeks. She did not know his date of birth or middle name but was okay with him being with her and her children. She never asked us if she was in trouble, if the male was in trouble, or the status of her kids.

We arrived at the district and took the female inside. The detectives exited the interview room just as we secured the female. The detectives told me that the little girl was on life support and that the male was going to be charged then with aggravated child abuse, and they would contact the state's attorney about applicable charges for the female once they were done with the interview. They requested that I transport the male suspect to central booking, which I gladly obliged.

A few minutes later, the detectives brought the male suspect out of the interview room. He exited the room with a defiant swagger and rigid posture until he turned and saw me. As soon as he saw me, he shrunk and averted his stare, just as he did at the scene. I smiled and instructed him to turn around so that I could secure him in handcuffs. The suspect was mushy, and I thought he had finally realized his situation's seriousness. My recruit and I searched and secured the suspect, and I went back inside to get the arrest affidavit.

The detectives were waiting on me and asked if I had done anything to the suspect while I was on the scene earlier. I was confused because I had done nothing more than usual when asking for information. I did not say anything to him other than what was necessary to obtain the vital information for the detectives. They explained that he was very stoic and defiant during the interview when they met him at the district. He was very proper and did not even ask for a lawyer. He was dismissive, as if they were wasting his time. They said he acted the same way until he turned and saw me in the hallway, then melted. I told them I noticed it, too, but it was not due to anything I said or did to him.

As I explained, this incident was like any other; nothing separated it from others I had responded to or assisted in. However, I now had the information that the female child was on life support. I had no idea how old she was, what happened, or any potential she may have had for recovery. Not to leave things undone, I now had the affidavit, the charging document, and I did not resist the temptation to read it.

I discovered that the little girl, our victim, was under the age of two, and her brother was four. The children were a nuisance to the suspect and mother and spent most of their time locked in the bathroom of this small efficiency, while their mother and the male suspect spent most of their time playing an online game or spending time with one another. Over several weeks, the children were malnourished and had been fed only protein shakes, which caused diarrhea in the young children, and they were left to sit in their filth for extended periods. The treatment, as you can imagine, would cause the children to cry, as was the case here. The male suspect, who was allegedly *trained* in martial arts, would lose his temper, and he would physically abuse the children. He was the one that wrote "Dumbass" on the little boy's forehead.

On the morning of the incident, the mother and male suspect were playing online, and the little girl apparently would not stop crying in the bathroom. So, this fucking animal took the little girl from the bathroom. Using his cupped hands, keeping his thumb and fingers bent and close together, he hit the little girl around her ears repeatedly. The little girl did not stop crying, so he swaddled her tiny body in a motel towel, placed her inside his *martial arts* gear bag, and zipped it up. Not satisfied with his work, he put the bag on the floor and used it as a backrest while he sat against her as he played his online game.

The effect of a grown man's weight on a confined and swaddled child acted in the same fashion as a boa constrictor. Every breath the little girl took, her body would compress under his weight, and her next breath would be less and less until she suffocated. The mother did nothing to stop him or protect her children at any time. Both children had been mistreated and tortured until one was rendered unconscious with no interference from their biological mother.

I knew that I would give my recruit the affidavit, and if I had been unprofessional at any point, my recruit would surely pick up on it, and it may have a bearing on the case. So, I remained, as always, professional. I do not believe I said a single word while the suspect was transported. We got him out of the car and walked him into booking.

We got back in the car at booking, and I asked my recruit if he wanted to go to the hospital. We were both curious about why the sergeant did not want me there. He immediately said yes, and off we went.

I have already explained that I always had a one-liner ready or straightforward saying that I would spout off occasionally. One was *"if one gets away, two have to pay."* Usually followed by, "We do not determine guilt or innocence; it is our job to balance the universe, *yin and yang.*" From time to time, these were used by recruits and later by deputies I worked with over the years; back to our story.

We arrived at All Children's Hospital and entered the pediatric intensive care unit. Before we go any further, I feel that it is necessary to point out my belief that the medical staff in pediatric intensive care are absolute angels. I cannot explain or understand what it takes for them to do their jobs for even a day. They are truly remarkable, and this visit was no exception.

As my recruit and I entered the floor, I could feel the tension in the air. It increased as we neared the nurse's station and found a literal wall of angry nurses greeting us. The charge nurse informed me that we would not take the little boy. I had no idea what she was talking about until she moved aside, and I saw the little boy from the incident scene sitting at the nurse's station. I almost did not recognize him. He was clean, free of the "dumbass" brand, surrounded by empty *Happy Meal* boxes and coloring books. Shockingly, he appeared like any other happy child. Now, with a full belly and a half dozen big sisters, this little boy was safer than he had been in quite some time. I quickly told the charge nurse that we responded to the incident scene and had already met the little boy. I told her the suspect was in jail, with the mother to follow by lunchtime, and we had no intention of taking him anywhere. We wanted to check in on the patient. This was the missing piece to our puzzle.

Luckily, the mood changed, and I sensed neither my recruit nor I were in danger. The nurse took us into the little girl's room, and I was unprepared for what we saw. This little girl was covered in leads connected to machines, and she had been intubated and connected to a ventilator. Through all of the medical apparatus, we could see the little girl. She had blonde hair, fair skin, and, by my judgment, extremely thin. Too thin, emaciated. Children under two usually have chubby little legs that stick out from the diaper, pull-up, or big kid pants. The thickest part of this little girl's thigh was thin enough for the nurse to wrap her fingers around with her index finger and thumb touching.

There was not a single area on her body that had not been bruised by the fucking animal we just dropped off at the jail.. Do you recall the cupping of the hands and striking the little girl's ears, trying to get her to stop crying? Her fair skin readily provided evidence of that trauma. Her cheeks, just in front of both ears, showed faint bruising. Behind her ears were four distinct bruises in an arc where the suspect's fingers impacted. This little girl had been broken, tortured, battered, and suffocated while the woman who birthed her watched without protest.

My face was tingling, and I was nauseous. I had a four-year-old and a two-year-old at home, and I left them sleeping soundly and safely in their beds. I asked the nurse what her prognosis was. She ran down the list of medical maladies, some of which were familiar sounding and others that did not sound promising. The last thing the nurse said stuck with me and rattled in my head still to this day. She sorrowfully said, "She's an angel now."

With that, I looked at my recruit, who was still standing at the foot of the tiny bed. Without breaking eye contact with the little girl, he resolutely asked, "Are you ready to balance the universe?" At that moment, all I could think was *fuck yes*.

My recruit and I left the hospital and returned to our zone after completing our reports. Due to the depth and complexity of this investigation, we were mostly done for the day, though our involvement was peripheral at best. We did not talk about the call.

Question #1: Why did the male suspect shrink at my

presence? In retrospect, I believe the suspect knew what he had done to her, but he did not know how much of that I knew when he first saw me. I can only assume by his shrinking reaction to my presence and his defiant behavior toward others that he knew I was the *Alpha* and had within me the capacity to take his life.

My sergeant was right not to send me to the hospital first. At that moment, bedside, and to this day I know, had I seen what this fucking animal had done to this little girl and later saw him sitting boldly on that stool, I would have kicked the stool from beneath him, buried my pistol to the breach in his mouth, and smiled as I sent him straight to hell. I think he felt that when he saw me, and he was right.

Question #2: Was he convicted? Yes, he was convicted of second-degree murder and sentenced to twenty years. He was sentenced in 2011 and has a prospective release date of 2026, less than the twenty-year sentence.

My thoughts here are not limited to this incident but the entire weekend. Adding that I had a recruit is essential because, as a trainer, I was responsible for ensuring my recruit was processing and adjusting to our experiences that weekend. I would have listened had he voiced concern, but neither of us did. I had an issue, obviously, with the volume and types of calls we had over this work cycle and should have thought more of the recruit's needs. I had a physical reaction to the scenes, was completely neutral about the thought of killing the male suspect, and was emotionally and physically worn by the end of Sunday. Still, I said nothing. The recruit and I maintained a professional relationship throughout the rest of my career, and we never spoke of this call or the weekend again.

My lesson here is that as *experienced* first responders, we should be more aware that everyone is different in their

Hiding in Plain Sight

capacity to experience and process trauma. Our first signal to check on one another should be any call that a non-responder would find challenging to deal with, followed by any noticeable changes in our partners.

I have found that being vulnerable and speaking about the effects of some of my experiences has also prompted others to speak up. I liken this to being in a class and having a question but not being willing to ask, fearing looking silly. You know someone else in the class has the same question, but neither of you wantt to be the one to ask. In this situation, as in mine, no one learns.

Chapter 16

Scene 9, I Never Knew Her Name

One of my regrets over the years was forgetting or never knowing the names of the people I had contact with. I need to explain what I mean here. If we met and I thought I would see you again, I would likely remember your name. If not, then it was left to chance. As with my general malaise about meeting new people, so was my eagerness to catalog every contact I had. Some are more memorable than others. Most fade or aren't worth remembering. I am unsure if this was a sign of losing empathy, becoming more apathetic, or compassion fatigue. I know that as a responder, you will contact scores of people daily, and maybe there are too many to keep track of. I went to or happened upon calls I regret not finding out more about before pressing on to the next one. One such call occurred at the end of a fourteen-hour off-duty job.

I was assigned to the bomb disposal team, and one of my duties was to conduct searches and sweeps and respond to suspicious packages during large venue gatherings. I was leaving Raymond James Stadium after a Tampa Bay Buccaneers game and took the back roads home to avoid being stuck in stadium traffic. This was the first time I took this route, and it just so happened that I made up the route as I went along. Luckily, I made all the lights except the large intersection at Dale Mabry Highway and Waters Avenue.

First, I should explain to non-law enforcement officers that a phenomenon occurs when you want to get home. Someone in traffic needs something. This is usually signaled by someone waving their hands like fools in the car next to you, trying to get your attention. The natural response to this is to say aloud, "*Faaaaaaaaaaaaaaaaaack*," while looking straight ahead and keeping your hands at 10 and 2. This never works, so you put on a large fake grin and roll down your window. Ninety-nine times out of one hundred, it's some asshole asking where Busch Gardens is or just wanting to thank you for your service.

This was the 100th time. I rolled down my window, and the passenger was frantic. She was asking where the hospital was, and I noticed she had something bundled in her arms. While processing the sights and sounds, I heard her say that her baby wasn't moving. Now, I knew the nearest hospital was a half mile south of us, slightly further than the nearest Fire Rescue station. No matter how good our dispatch and Fire Rescue were, we would be at the hospital before they arrived. So, I hit the lights and said follow me. We went south on Dale Mabry; they were right on my bumper. We were so close to the hospital that I barely had time to notify the dispatchers of what I had and where I was going before we arrived.

Screeching to a halt in front of the ER, I took the limp baby in my arms and noticed she was not breathing. This little girl fit on my arm like the resuscitation dolls we use for pediatric CPR training. Resting on my forearm, I started compressions while running into the ER, Mom and Dad in tow. I was in my utility uniform and a bomb squad t-shirt. I was not readily identifiable as a law enforcement officer, other than the pistol on my thigh; security initially stirred when I hit the door to go back into the ER.

I cleared the doors while delivering compressions and brought the nurses and doctor up to speed. The nurse scooped the baby from my arms, and their team went to work. Deputies in the area came to the hospital after hearing the radio traffic. For some reason, they thought I was there with my child, so I quickly cleared up the confusion.

After the commotion, I overheard the baby's mother telling a nurse that the little girl had a fever, and she gave her a children's medication commonly used to break a fever; the baby had an adverse reaction and then stopped responding after a few minutes. They were new to the area and did not know where the nearest hospital was, and they saw me as I stopped at the light. After that, I just left. I want to believe the baby survived, but I could not attest to that. I never asked her name.

In retrospect, I believe I left because I did not want to know. I thought wondering and hoping she survived and lived happily ever after was better than knowing the alternative. To some degree, I was right, but if I had known one way or the other, this story would not have made it into the book. More importantly, I would not have carried this question around for twelve years.

The lesson I found here was not that it was better to know or not know, but the broader lesson that avoidance and denial will only delay the inevitable truth. There will be a reckoning; someday, you must revisit the memory and sort it out.

Chapter 17

Scene 10, The Sound and The Screaming Eagle

A few sounds are immediately recognizable to some veterans and first responders. Some sounds are more familiar than others, but if heard only once, they are unmistakable. Among this list may be gunshots-*incoming vs. outgoing,* a scream of terror, agonal breathing or the last exhale, and a person getting a chest tube without anesthesia. These may affect people in very different ways. The response to these sounds may be an automatic call to action or a flinch reaction in response to the latter.

There is one sound that is unmistakable and needs no context. It is the only sound in the world like it, not mimicked by anything I have ever heard in nature. One that tears pieces from your soul, fracturing every fiber in your being. In fairness, it is not only the sound but the association of the sound to the pain and emotion that causes it to be generated. It is the sound a mother makes when she finds out one of her children is dead. It is not a cry or scream but an inconsolable wail, like a banshee. It is a sound that tears your heart in half and leaves you empty.

The Screaming Eagle

As a supervisor, I routinely responded to death investigations to ensure nothing was missed and all notifications had been made. I would generally arrive just after the initial responding deputies and assist in setting work priorities, which in many instances initially involved clearing the area and scene preservation. This call was similar to many death investigations but struck me differently.

I arrived on the scene, and several deputies were already there. I was told by one of the deputies on the scene that the deceased was in the living room and had a single gunshot wound to the side of the head, which appeared to have been self-inflicted. He said he was signal 7, *the signal code we use for "deceased."*

I walked into the one-bedroom apartment and asked if it had been cleared. Seldom missing an opportunity to teach and provide guidance, we cleared the small apartment to ensure no other occupants were present.

The apartment's layout was pretty straightforward. Everything was in place; there were no signs of forced entry or a struggle. We were confident no one else was inside, and the deceased appeared to have lived alone. I noticed several things that struck me unrelated to the incident, just things that have stuck with me. These things left me thinking, even to this day, more than twelve years later.

First, the dining area to my right as I entered. There was a bookshelf in the room. A MICH helmet with a Surefire helmet light and a Surefire 9V flashlight rested on it. These were military-issued and still had the faint stain of dust matted in the helmet's texture and the lights' crevices. His bedroom was neat, the bed was made, and all the shoes were lined up *dress right dress.* He had some civilian clothes hanging in his closet, but most hanging garments were multicam fatigues and a set of Army dress blues. The patches were immediately recognized- the *Screaming Eagle.* I remember shuttering at first and then taking a deep breath.

Then, to the main room. I stood in the sitting area at the feet of our decedent, who was seated on the floor. He was a young man in his very early twenties. He was fully dressed, with an Xbox controller and Glock pistol sitting to his right. He was gone.

I had unanswered questions, like where this kid's teammates were, where the help was for him, where his family was, and why he had to die alone or at all. As I stood there, I started thinking about what the deputy said to me when I arrived, signal 7. Although I have said and heard "signal 7" countless times, this was the first time I contemplated the sterility and matter-of-fact nature in which cops describe someone's death. The description of all they were, how they lived, and how they died had been reduced to two simple words: Signal Seven.

Deep in this thought, I was surprised and unprepared for what would come next. There was a knock at the door. It was late in the evening and too early for detectives. *Shit, I hope it's not a guest.* It was worse. The decedent's brother and mother were at the door. One of my deputies called and asked me to step out with him. I walked out, and both of them stared at me. It is never a good sign that the police are at anyone's house. The brother was stoic and knew what was coming. Mom was in shock. Her expression was completely vacant, hoping for the best but knowing what was coming. After dozens of notifications, I still had not perfected or polished my delivery. How does one get good at telling someone a loved one is dead? I took her hand in mine, and before I said anything, she dropped to her knees. This was not the first time I had heard the sound, but this one stuck with me. If you have been unfortunate enough to hear it, or worse, make it, you understand, and I am truly sorry.

The unfortunate thing that I have discovered about trauma, or at least my experiences with trauma, is that when you avoid it, it sticks around until it is replaced by or eclipsed by something even more fucked up. This sound of her scream rattled in my head until, like all the others, it was replaced by something else. It then becomes a memory of an event that we compartmentalize and put in a box. Shoved way down, it sits loaded like a fucking Jack in the Box. I have never spoken of this to anyone.

Chapter 18

Scene 11, A Simple Marker and Indelible Mark.

We join this scene in the middle to close out the scene that launched the book. You may recall it included a young girl under a white sheet and me walking toward an unknowing and intent father.

I looked at the younger deputy, my back to the now-gathering crowd; she looked beyond me and said she would stay with the girl if I would deal with Dad. Confused by her reply, I turned and saw a man crumbling emotionally and moving as quickly as he could toward his daughter, who was now lying under a white sheet.

The look on his face was the look of indescribable pain. As he got closer, I think he realized at the same time I did that I was the only thing standing between him and his little girl. I had no idea what I was going to say or do. I did know that, were I in his position, what it would take to prevent me from getting to my little girl and that I would not be enough. To that point in my professional life, I had never been pushed, punched, kicked, or even touched by anyone who had the intent to harm me. I was able to de-escalate or physically end any confrontation before one began. But at that moment, I believed this man was going to beat my ass, and I was going to let him.

We met face to face, and he told me to move. I put my hands in front of me and asked him to stop and listen to me. Oddly, he did. I told him that I was a father too, and I had no idea what he must be feeling at that moment, but it was taking everything I had in me to keep *my shit* together. I asked when the last time he saw his daughter was. He said that morning before he left for work. I asked if she was smiling, and he said that she was. I told him, remember that. He broke down. He started collapsing in the grass, and I hugged her father. I am unsure which of us was holding who up, but there we were.

I told him there was nothing we could do at this point, but I promised I would not leave his side, and when the time came, I would go with him to see his daughter. Neither of us had any fight left, and he accepted my offer. I stood on the side of Interstate 75 with the family, narrating the process while the troopers took measurements and pictures. The medical examiner arrived, and I checked in, asking that the family be allowed to come over before they removed her from the scene. I went back and spoke to the family and told them that the medical examiner would come and get us when it was time. Her father thanked me for staying with them and said I could leave; he wanted to handle this. I knew that he wanted to face this with his family, and I was quietly relieved I did not have to go back and bear further witness to their life-altering event.

Luckily, and for reasons we will get into later, I had opportunities to empty the proverbial bucket of trauma before this scene. However, this was a lot, and for the first time, I parked under a tree and made a video on my phone to capture my feelings. My reaction was a mixture of sadness and rage; sadness for apparent reasons, but rage and confusion as to *why* this tragedy had to happen in the first place.

I finished the video and went back to the district office for lunch. I was late for lunch, and as luck would have it, the young deputy with me on the crash scene was in the break room eating lunch.

She was reticent, and her gaze was different than it had been at the beginning of the shift. Older, somehow wiser, but puzzled. She was still processing the scene in her head. I asked if she wanted to talk about it, and she appeared surprised that I asked. She thanked me for my concern, but it was still too fresh for us to assign meaningful words. She asked me what I had said to the father, and I told her the truth. I told her I shared with the father that I was scared and confused, too, but I would stay with him until it was done. She shared with me her vantage point and remarked that no one else could have done what I did. In reflection, and now in the white space offered by time and distance, I guess I was there specifically for that reason.

I spoke with Michelle about the event late that night. Talking about calls was something I stopped doing years prior, thinking that I was sparing her from the trauma I had experienced. Unfortunately, I wore each event like a shirt. I knew what happened at each event, and in my silence, she was left to imagine what I had experienced. In retrospect, I don't know if that was tougher on her than knowing. Nevertheless, I shared this event because I was grateful that I was there for the father and that I had recognized a co-worker in need. This was growth for me.

In the days after, I found the young girl's father's Facebook page and would occasionally check it. I wanted to see how he was doing without making my presence known or having to muster the courage to face him again. Every night for the following year, he posted to her page. He told her about his day, told her a sweet story, and said good night.

This event is vital to my journey for many reasons, but none more significant than it was the first event that I noticed someone had a problem in the *after*, and I asked them if they wanted help. This was also the first event in my 27-year professional life that I consciously dwelled on until I dealt with it. I would traverse my zone using Interstate 75 several times a day and would consciously look at the tree and the then-new memorial placed by her family on the spot where she died.

On long weekends with my family, we would travel that section of Interstate 75, and every time I found it, I would look at the memorial when we passed it. As if acknowledging it had become an addiction, something I had no control over. Michelle knew what I was doing and could feel me winding up as we got closer and would hold my hand.

More than a year had passed since the crash, and I received a transfer back to the district where I had spent most of my career. I had a choice on my last day in the old zone. I can face her and put this to rest or transfer out of the zone and let it linger. Deep down, we hold onto these events and faces because, for some unexplained reason, we do not want to forget. I am unsure if we don't seek respite because we are punishing ourselves or if we think we must stay *hardened* to the effects of those still to come.

On my last day in the zone, I drove to roughly the same spot I parked on the shoulder the day of the crash. I walked through the tall grass to the memorial and had a conversation. I knew there was nothing I could have done to have influenced her survivability, but I did finally permit myself to let it go. I have not been drawn to look at the memorial since, and I no longer feel anxiety building as we drive that stretch of road. I was done keeping company with ghosts, at least this one.

Chapter 19

Leadership Opportunities

Throughout my career, I would be forced to endure poor leadership at the hands of Martinets, narcissists, cowards, and weak men. I experienced them all and felt the impact of their management styles firsthand. Despite these experiences, I was mindful that man is human and, as such, is corruptible. Being loyal to a person will ultimately leave you with a decision when they decide to act on something you may disagree with- to follow or retreat. Early on, I adopted the military mindset to mitigate this potential issue. I remained loyal to the ideals that brought me to the profession, the sheriff's office, and supported the billet regardless of who filled it.

The profession, the office, and the title are in and of themselves not corruptible. It is the actions of the people in them that bring corruption. If I agreed in principle with the person in the billet, my life would be easy. If I did not, I would need to determine if it was a matter of style or an example of poor leadership. I could deal with style, but poor leadership posed some problems. I learned early to speak truth to power and manage up. I did not always do it tactfully, but I got my point across. Staying loyal to my purpose and profession led me to do great things professionally.

Leadership Can Be Learned

As a young Airman, I was fortunate to have been mentored by some outstanding airmen early on. They took me in and invested in me. They understood interdependence and knew intuitively that my success meant our success. I learned what good leadership looked like. I could take their positive examples and discern them from the poor examples.

I built my leadership style on what felt right and the mounting list of things not to do. As a young non-commissioned officer, I tested my leadership theories and, more importantly, learned from the leadership examples set by the *operators*, NCOs, and officers I was exposed to during my last ten years in the Air Force. I was mentored by quiet and accomplished men and women who demonstrated selfless leadership and commitment to one another and the mission. I was given insight into higher-level decision-making processes and the 10,000-foot view. Trust and competence were valued most in this atmosphere.

I witnessed how leadership drives the culture of any organization, regardless of size. A single example of good leadership and demonstrating the standard of behavior can turn the tide on an entire company. Conversely, toxic leadership, or a culture in which people do not feel valued or safe, is destined for corruption and collapse.

I always felt that being an example for others to follow was more impactful than telling someone the standard. Being the example provided a clear picture and ensured that there was never a question about what was acceptable; it endeared me to those I worked for and my troops and inspired others to raise their game.

I quickly found that being an example drew hard stares from those I considered less than capable of meeting the standard. My first obvious example of this came when I was a recruit class coordinator in the training division. Instead of drinking coffee while the recruits were getting smoked during PT, I would PT with them. Not as the leader or instructor but at the back of the line. When they ran, I ran. When they pushed, I pushed. I would visit the range when they were training and shoot with them. I grabbed a bucket first when it was time to pick up brass. I was at work before them and there after they left. This was something that no other coordinator or instructor was doing at the time, and I drew the ire of my co-workers, as well as from the martinet sergeant, who believed that I was blurring the lines between superior and subordinate.

Despite the cost, the reward for my efforts was an entire class of recruits who knew what good leadership looked like. When they rose to that position, many of whom eventually did, they would have a template. The benefits to me were just as meaningful. PT with the class kept me in physical shape and sent a message that physical fitness was necessary regardless of where one was in one's career. The moments spent with the recruits also allowed me to get to know each of them better.

Initially, I wanted to be in a leadership position to right all the wrongs I had experienced at the hands of poor leadership. More importantly, I wanted to be in a position to help younger deputies achieve whatever goals they were working toward; having the positional ability to impact the lives of those like-minded hard chargers positively was the greatest joy and privilege of leadership. Sharp troops who felt valued and safe contributed to the overall health and future of the organization.

I looked to make every opportunity a win-win. I towed the company line, believed in it, and acted in the organization's and my troops' best interests. This was easy because I sincerely believed in the profession, the organization, and my troops that every decision and action aligned with my personal beliefs. I was a living part of the organizational machine. I did these things in earnest.

The shaved-head hard charger brand got me to the edge of promotion and placed me front and center, apart from my peers. I was promoted to corporal and was moved into positions to supplant or support weak supervisors or provide stronger leadership wherever needed. I was used as an enforcer and problem solver. I must be clear: I was not a paper hanger, and my presence and actions led people to improve.

I had been *passed over* for promotion to sergeant for several years. I finally found someone with enough character to have a hard conversation with me and give honest and constructive feedback. I was told that I give the perception that I am rigid and inflexible and intimidate other supervisors. The attributes that suited me for their use as an enforcer were now a weakness. I replied that someone's lack of self-esteem was not my problem. He smiled as if I had just confirmed his observation.

In response to his candor and mentorship, I worked in earnest to rebrand. I let my hair grow out and bought a comb. I parted my hair to the side, which made me appear more approachable. I changed nothing else. I was noticed for my intellect and leadership attributes within months. I was soon promoted to sergeant and, within two years, to lieutenant. I was once again assigned to sections to supplant weak supervisors and provide stronger leadership, but I was still the enforcer and problem solver. I guess perception is reality.

I led by example and from the front. I did not tolerate laziness, cowardice, or liars. These were well-known facts, and anyone with those traits stayed well clear of my path. If one of my troops demonstrated a deficiency in work, decision-making, or character, I would first weigh my actions by looking in the mirror. Where was my culpability? Did I fail to demonstrate the standard? Where did I need to shore up my game? Or was this an inability or refusal to meet the standard? Inability and refusal are different. If someone gave their best effort and was simply a C *student,* I was satisfied that they were giving their best, and I would contribute what I could to their success. If they were an A *student* simply coasting and giving C *student* work, then they would be in line for an uncomfortable conversation. But it always began with me.

When making decisions, I always balanced the organization's needs with finding value in the solution—value for the employee, my supervisors, and the organization. Building *leadership capital* is a term I heard used by Jocko Willink years into my leadership tenure. As he explained, it was difficult to build and easy to lose. Building leadership capital cost me nothing, no more than what I was already doing or capable of doing. As a lieutenant, tracking with K9, being the shield man, or even kicking in a door to retrieve a barricaded subject was not outside of the norm for me. A good foot chase and a resist was always on my list of *to-dos* should the opportunity arise.

I was in a position where I could improve the lives of those I worked for (my subordinates), which also fed my sense of value. The investment of my time and talents in my personnel paid dividends. They knew what leadership looked like, and I felt great about being *that guy.*

As with land navigation, one step to the right or left of

azimuth is imperceptible initially, but given enough distance, you will be far off course, possibly even lost. The same holds true in life. In 2015, I left the path of my purpose. It did not seem relevant then, but eventually, it took me off my path altogether, leaving me lost. I became loyal to a person rather than a group of people with positional authority. They made me feel valued and put me in positions to perform and highlight my talents. I was promoted in 2016 due to my continued hard work and positive results, partly due to their provision of a stage and opportunity to show my abilities. I felt important, like I had graduated from the kid's table, as if I were now somehow anointed and counted among trusted advisors. I went where they told me and did the things that they suggested I do. I was comfortable having hard conversations and holding people accountable. They positioned me in places they felt needed improvement. I was a change agent, one of their enforcers.

    I outperformed my predecessors at every turn. With the help and guidance of a strong lieutenant, I became adept at *managing up*. I had the bosses' confidence, and I was in their counsel. I soon found that their approval, particularly the command staff, fed my ego and gave me a sense of importance. More so than my own validation. The dopamine and oxytocin released from giving or receiving an atta boy replaced warm hugs. I found my worth here. I wanted to be important and useful, but not where it mattered most.

Chapter 20

My Drive and the Cost

"Whoever fights monsters should see to it that in the process, he does not become a monster. And if you gaze long enough into an abyss, the abyss will gaze back into you."

— Friedrich Nietzsche

Michelle and I were either dating, engaged, or married throughout my career. She was present for the last ten years of my military service and all twenty-five years in law enforcement. She dealt with deployments, callouts, hurricane details, six weeks of bomb school while she was pregnant with our son, and midnight shifts with small children. She was, for all intents and purposes, a single mom. She, and later our children, bore the brunt of my career, my absence, and my emotional isolation. It was not until after I broke and, more importantly, began to heal that I realized this.

I was selfish in everything I did, and the half-truth masked every decision. I was pushing hard for more opportunities to eventually get promoted, make more money, get off the road, and better support my family. *Fill in the blank* with whatever you need to sell the idea to yourself or your family. Although these benefits were a byproduct of hard work, they were never my motivation. I pushed harder because I wanted to be the best, and I wanted everyone to know it without me ever having to say a word. Soon, this drive led me to believe this was what gave me worth; this made me important. Their quiet admiration of my contributions to the machine fed me.

In time, this turned into a crippling fear of failure or seemingly falling short of the expectations of those who entrusted me with the job. This ensured that I was on top of everything, on time, top-notch, every time. I worked hard and became known as the field training expert, the bomb guy, the WMD guy, the terrorism guy, and the emergency management guy. I was consistent and dependable. Given a task, the tasker never had to touch it again. Give me Y to execute, and Y was executed. A troubled recruit salvaged, a bomb callout with a quiet resolution, and hurricane responses planned and executed were all the things that fed me but ultimately did not fill me.

An attaboy would carry me a long way. The highs were very high, and conversely, a terse word or my perception of falling out of favor would send me into a deep spiral. The lows were just as extreme as the highs. I have found that depending so profoundly on your profession or the fickle opinions of others leaves you vulnerable to the changing winds. Any change in the wind could leave you with an overrated sense of self or, just as dangerous, a feeling of betrayal. I had the unrealistic expectation that someday, the profession or the organization would love me back.

In 2015, I trusted people in positions of authority to decide where I was best suited and would most serve the organization.

I relied on their opinions and metrics of success. I was chasing a moving target. How would I know when I became successful? Was it money, rank, admiration? Chasing a subjective end state or a goal line determined by someone else leaves you rudderless, searching, and never fulfilling your purpose. I did not set any personal or professional boundaries and sought more opportunities. No matter how far outside my wheelhouse or ability, I never said no to the bosses. I saw each challenge as an opportunity to rise to the occasion. Looking back on a job well done, I realized that I had received the conditional admiration of those bosses, which fed my ego and led me to feel successful. In the end, this was empty and fruitless. I thought I was being useful, but I was just used.

I later learned this is referred to as the ambition of shame. In short, I was driven to successful outcomes due to my fear of letting someone down, forming my persona into something I believed they wanted to see instead of fulfilling my purpose. This stemmed from the shame and guilt I carried away from time with my teammates. I let them down; I failed them. I never wanted to feel that again, so I smashed through every obstacle, refusing to stop.

Tying my identity to my profession, this persona, was a dangerous game. There was no off-ramp and no rest. I was always driving forward and outworking or outpacing my peers. There was nothing more important to me than being able to be *the guy* when the guy was needed. Always on the door or the shield, the constant need to be the number one on a bomb callout, the guy that could fix the administrative problem or the training deficiency. I wanted to be the *In Case of ____ Break Glass* option. No successful end state, lack of professional boundaries, and unwisely picking priorities left only filling that open blank with things that could be done professionally and, quite frankly, could have been accomplished by a few others. I was never the *In Case Dad* or *Husband Break Glass* options, and I would later pay a hefty price.

The Cost

From the onset of my career, I was driven by passion and purpose. I strayed from the path slowly, almost imperceptibly, and became overinvested and immersed, so much so that I allowed my professional abilities and identity to define my self-worth and actual identity. I was serious about my role and profession but took myself too seriously. Fear of failure or letting someone down, ego, and the opinions of others fueled my drive to fulfill my purpose. Doug was fused and lost in Deputy White, and I allowed it to influence and take precedence over being present for my family and, toward the end of my career, living for my purpose.

These symptoms did not appear all at once, and slight changes occurred over time. Trying to put a time stamp on when I became unhealthy is challenging to do because these events happened over time, and my body adapted. The allostatic load I was under was extreme and unrelenting. My threshold was pushed daily, and with each incident, my baseline changed. I adapted and became used to the new normal. It was also difficult to identify the changes using the members of my circles as a litmus test. Military or civilian, we were all experiencing the same events in real-time at the same time. Regardless of the impact of a single event, or perhaps the chronic and acute exposure to trauma, in effect, we were made sick by the same poison at a similar rate. To each other, we were perfectly normal.

Compounding issues, most first responders live and work in

the same communities. This is a lifelong roller coaster of fight or flight. Adrenaline dumps and tragedy. Days off do not provide enough time to rest, and you take hypervigilance on vacation. There is no hiding from it. Every corner and every street had a story. In the beginning and over time, hypervigilance, depression and anxiety, anger, nightmare and apnea-induced sleep disturbances, and apathy joined together, producing a powder keg with a slow-burning fuse.

I first noticed faint signs of my issues in October 2006. I was thirty-three years old and in solid physical shape. I was assigned to the training division and had grand visions of the wonderful things that I and my recruit class would accomplish. I was driven to ensure that I dedicated every effort to imparting skills and my experiences to the class members, so much so that almost everything else became background noise.

I had moments of clarity during this time, but they did not sway me from my mission. I recall when I realized I was missing out on my family. I was at the range with the class. It was late, easily an hour before I got home. It was Halloween, and my daughter was not yet two. Michelle called me and asked if I was on the way home. I had just left the range, and she told me they were wrapping up a trick-or-treating in the neighborhood and that she would keep our daughter in costume so I could see her. I got home after dark, about an hour after Michelle and I had spoken. I pulled into the driveway, and an exhausted miniature Snow White awaited me. She was adorable and could barely keep her eyes open. I regretted not being there but thought I was working toward the greater good, being there for my troops. I knew I was wrong, but I used the experience to drive harder, reminding myself what I had sacrificed for the class's success. This trend would continue for the greater part of my career.

I was promoted to corporal in July of 2010. I was a new supervisor on the midnight shift and was quickly reminded that working twelve-hour night shifts was the great equalizer. Driving hard professionally, and the unresolved chronic and acute trauma I had experienced throughout my career had been chasing me for years by this point. Lack of sleep magnified the issues and made them harder to control. I had become more brooding and would ruminate on events longer than in the past, to the point where it would keep me awake. Though I became more aware that I was having issues, I did not have a name for it yet.

Hypervigilance

I am relatively confident that most cops have heard the phrase: *be courteous, professional, and have a plan to kill everyone you meet.* This was said tongue in cheek; the reality is that not everyone you come in contact with is a threat or trying to kill you. These phrases, experiences on the road, and little to no time to reset or find balance before returning to shift are recipes for disaster.

If you are in law enforcement or have spent an amount of time as a protector, be it a community, other soldiers, or your family, ask this simple question. When was the last time you were in a public place and sat with your back to the door? I bet you know the location of every door, make eye contact with each person who enters, and quickly determine *threat/no threat* while trying to decide if you should get an appetizer. I have been doing things for the past 30 years. I was to the point that when the meal was done, I was ready for the bill and then to leave. There was no time for dessert. I would get more anxious if the kids wanted a scoop of ice cream. Dining in restaurants and just being in large public places left me exhausted. Anxiety would turn into anger, which would lead me to isolate myself from everyone else. The unfortunate side effect was that my avoidance and isolation led to me isolating my family from these experiences.

I was always on edge. I was always at 98 out of 100. When triggered by anything I perceived as a threat or a reminder of certain events, I felt a visceral reaction. My default was anger and reaction, and I was immediately ready for a fight. In traffic, I would visualize an event and outcome and find that I had driven a distance and had no idea how I had gotten there. I would give hard stares to anyone who made eye contact with me. I did not shy away from the notion of physical confrontation, and sometimes, I may have invited it.

I was on a years-long rollercoaster of hypervigilance. My respite was inside my home, entertaining myself with mindless activities like sitting on the couch or playing video games. Avoiding crowds and not wanting to meet new people took a toll on my family. I was always ready for a fight and could not relax in a crowd. I was standoffish, generally unfriendly, and would even get amped up at Disney World. I just wanted peace. It was not until recently that I learned that hypervigilance is a neurological change. One that you do not have control over. It is automatic and your body's means of keeping you alive. Being in that state for so long allows for habituation; in other words, you get used to it, and it becomes the baseline. Ninety-eight out of one hundred had become the new base.

Avoidance

I avoided the 800-pound gorilla in the room. I minimized or denied the issues I was having even though the symptoms were apparent to me and hidden from others. Avoiding the issues meant that I did not have to confront them—anxiety, depression, sleep disturbances, and, oddly enough, chronic pain. Not addressing the root issues as they arose or watering them down only allowed them to grow larger. Leading later to shame, regret, and anger.

Dark humor or an inappropriate reaction to trauma triggers became part of the routine. Topics of *everyday* conversation that would leave the average civilian with a sense of unease and sleepless nights were part and parcel of the job. Dark humor was a coping mechanism that helped break the tension of traumatic or stressful events. Telling a joke or making light of a tragic situation released some tension but also sent a message that everyone else was *okay* or *fine*. People were joking, so that must mean something is wrong with me if I have an issue with it.

Another form of avoidance was staying away from things that negatively affected me, such as the gas station my friend visited just hours before he died in the breezeway of the grocery store I shop at, the street my shootout occurred on, songs that reminded me of something or someone, and people and crowds in general.

Isolation

The profession itself isolates you, either by design or accident. As a younger law enforcement officer, my circle consisted of my squad mates, who were roughly the same age. I did not associate with anyone I felt was *less than*. In other words, someone who should have taken the profession more seriously. I surrounded myself with meat eaters and go-getters—people who trained and were prepared for their careers. We shared a competitive drive to be the best. Our work experiences were similar as we all worked together. We understood each other and always had something to talk about. Unfortunately, the subject was always work.

Trying to broaden the circle was difficult due to shift work. Finding non-coworkers leading professional grown-up lives to hang out with on a Tuesday morning was difficult. So, you either did co-worker stuff or just went solo. Going the co-worker route always meant you would speak about work or the profession at large.

Isolating with co-workers may seem like building Esprit de Corps or investing in a friendship, and I am sure this may happen on occasion. Still, in retrospect, I found that I surrounded myself with people similar to me, and the things we would speak about were not regular topics. It would be normal to sit over breakfast and coffee and talk candidly about traffic fatalities or other horrific scenes in detail, sprinkling in graveyard humor. Common speaking points were topics that would shock the senses of any healthy person. On occasion, these conversations almost seemed to spiral into a childish game of *one-upmanship* or *no shit; there I was*. This was not healthy.

Being a service member or responder also has unfortunate social side effects. When you are in a group of non-responders or non-service members, you seem to be a novelty to those who have not had your experiences. Going to any gathering as a cop, you would most assuredly hear something like, "Hide the booze; the *cops are here*." "*Hey (fill in the name), they're here for you."* Or be surrounded by people who want to ask stupid shit like, *have you ever shot anyone* or *tell me about the worst call you have been on.*

In comparison, an insurance salesperson or dentist goes to a gathering, and they are just whatever their fucking names are. No one says dumb shit or asks nonsensical questions, wanting you to shock them by peeling back your trauma or someone else's. These interactions led me to stay away from gatherings or only seek company in groups where these questions would not be asked, which were once again co-workers or veterans.

Isolation, simply tuning out, closed my eyes to my culpability in my marriage's troubles. We were not communicating as spouses, and I took no active role in decision-making or spending time with my family. I resented her decisions without my input when, in fairness, I did not avail myself emotionally and did not want to make any decisions. I was wholly disengaged. I took everything as an insult.

There was a point when our relationship was sterile as if we were running a business. It was very transactional and almost guided by a task list. Michelle would make comments that she felt as if she were all alone, and these comments offended me as I saw them as dismissive of my hard work, as if I were not doing my part to provide for her and the kids. My perception of the comments was that they were offensive when, in fact, her comment was accurate and a veiled request for help, which I was deaf to. Years later, I would realize this on my own and admit to my shortcomings in these instances. After these conversations, and in true fashion, Michelle would absolve me of my guilt and shame from these shortfalls. She saw these conversations as signs of my growth and recovery and her validation of what she had felt during those times.

Lacking appreciation and gratitude for her contributions

and my taking offense to her observations of my disengaged behavior sent me further into depression, which unfortunately presented itself as anger and negative self-beliefs. I was quick to anger at the most minor issues. I found that I would react rather than respond to stimuli. Quick-tempered and quick to act and speak to my children certainly painted me as a bad guy. My entire family was walking on eggshells so they wouldn't upset me. I was the sleeping monster and would not realize this until years later. Ultimately, hypervigilance, compassion fatigue, and avoidance led me to seek peace in being alone and isolated.

Depression

Again, the lows were as extreme as the highs. There were instances where I would wake up and sit quietly in a dark room all day until I heard the garage door open, signaling someone was home. I would spring into action and pretend as if I had done something during the past eight hours. I stopped training or leaving the house and began comfort eating. My life had become joyless, and I only sought to be alone. I became hopeless.

Sleep Disturbances

I was on midnight shifts as a young airman and later as a newer deputy. As I aged, midnight shifts became more challenging to manage. My circadian rhythm was off, and I had difficulty falling asleep and even staying asleep beyond three or four hours. Regardless of my assigned shift, Michelle voiced concerns about my snoring, gasping, or stopping breathing altogether for years. Her concerns led me to have a sleep study done when I was about thirty-five years old. The sleep study results were concerning, but the doctor said I did not meet the threshold for sleep apnea because I did not stop breathing *enough* times per hour. I dismissed the issues as sinuses or a nightmare.

My sleep disturbances were magnified when I was assigned to midnight shifts. I was assigned to a district patrol platoon when I was promoted to corporal in 2010 and as an acting sergeant in 2013. After a four-year break on the day shift as a supervisor and a sergeant in a support division, I was promoted to lieutenant in 2018.

Newly promoted, I was assigned to a midnight shift platoon. Despite my ongoing sleep issues, I was getting what I thought was sufficient rest while assigned to day shift positions. However, back on midnights, my sleep quickly became more fragmented, and I could only sleep for about two to three hours at a time. On most occasions, I could not fall back to sleep. On rare occasions, I could get a quick nap before my shift. This lack of sleep caught up to me quickly. Insufficient sleep, fed by my other symptoms, created a doom loop where they supported each other. Exhaustion, irritability, brain fog, and more frequent migraines joined the cast of characters. It affected my motivation and ability to control the emotions I had avoided and tried to outrun for years. I found that without sleep, the things that you are generally able to manage become unmanageable. No sleep, stress, a flood of emotions from past traumas, and my perceived inability to maintain led me deeper into depression. The loop continued.

Apathy

Shift work and social awkwardness or novelty certainly do not help; these were just the beginning stages for me. As time went on, I would view civilians as *nasty* or *sheep*. Incapable of helping themselves or completely unaware, with no situational awareness. In retrospect, this viewpoint began when I was on active duty and was enforced over time. Responding to scores of events where you had to come to their rescue or sort out some situations in which they were the *victim* brought on by years of their bad decisions only deepened my ability to dismiss their troubles as trivial and self-inflicted, leaving me the thought of *fuck that guy* or *he had it coming*. Viewing people in this way generally leads to a point when they become dehumanized because of my inability to reset empathy or through compassion fatigue, where I physiologically and emotionally cannot take on their issues.

I am aware that there are actual victims in this world, people in the wrong place at the wrong time, and single-event tragedies can turn people's lives in an instant. I am not speaking of them. I am speaking of the people and places that you and everyone you work with are familiar with. The guy you arrested for domestic violence four times and was never convicted because the victim refuses to testify but will call you again when he gets drunk or rough. My favorite is the couple that has been married or together for five years yet do not know each other's middle name, age, or date of birth. There comes a point when continuing to help those who do not want help becomes seemingly pointless. This is a dangerous position for a first responder. Over time, my patience for people wore thin. A few days off here and there were not enough to reset, so disconnecting was easier.

Chapter 21

The Beginning of the End

My promotion to lieutenant in 2018 was the pinnacle of my professional achievements. It was the most significant opportunity to make a broad and positive impact in a leadership role, and I felt capable of performing any task before me. I reported to a district where I had spent much of my career. I was surrounded by solid leadership and great supporting supervisors, and my reputation ensured that many issues had sorted themselves out before I arrived. I set the tone and expectations for the platoon. I was very active and engaged with my deputies. My platoon enjoyed great success due to their hard work and the dedication of their supervisors.

After a few months on the night shift, I was reminded that midnights were the great equalizer. By April 2019, a combination of the weight of responsibility for twenty-eight souls, nearly twenty years of unresolved accumulated chronic trauma, and my inability to regulate my sleep provided me with an express ticket to burnout and beyond. Between April 2019 and November 2019, I slept an average of one and a half to three hours a day, on days off and on. I would be lucky on some days to fall asleep from exhaustion and nap for an hour or two before my shift, but that was often not the case.

Exhausted, I quickly found that life's happenings that were manageable, or I thought I was managing well, began slipping. I became much more aware of the stress I was encountering. It became more and more apparent that what I was experiencing was not situational or seasonal depression but the more significant signs and symptoms of PTS. These signs and symptoms were present for years, but I did not recognize them for what they were. Instead, I viewed each symptom individually; I did not connect one with the other. More importantly, I refused to speak to anyone about them.

As a supervisor, I would have squad and platoon meetings and always included a speech about how *it's okay not to be okay*. Later, when I became vocal about my struggle with PTS, one of my closest workmates and a supervisor who had worked with me for years asked if I had those conversations with the squads and platoon because I was looking for permission to get help myself. Or, if I thought I was alone? He was correct on both of his theories. He confided in me that he had hoped for the same outcome when I would have those conversations. Though I was sincere in my efforts and wanted my deputies to get help if needed, I remained the biggest hypocrite in the room.

Everything was falling apart at home, and it was all I could do to keep myself afloat at work. As the months progressed, I made more mistakes in my priorities. Prioritizing my health and getting help for any issues was not on the list. I began task shedding, getting rid of anything unnecessary for day-to-day survival. I was trying to be functional for work and for my family. You read the last sentence correctly-work was before family. The wheels were coming off, and I did not even acknowledge the severity of the potential impact. I just kept driving on.

I never missed one of the kids' functions at home, even if it meant I was in uniform in the back of the auditorium or behind the dugout. The house was always clean, laundry was done, and dinner was ready whenever the family arrived. Writing these last two sentences made me realize that only the first mattered. Being present was the big want. Although I was there physically, I was not present and had not been for years.

Before burning out at work, I quickly completed administrative and operational tasks. I was the accountability and details guy, and nothing was ever missed. I was engaged and active at work. By September 2019, my administrative tasks were all but disregarded. They were often put together just before the deadline and not representative of my best work. I spent most days at home in a dark room while the family was at school or work. I stopped training or exercising altogether and just existed. I was hopeless, and I hated myself.

During the Spring of 2019, I spoke with my leadership and vaguely informed them that I was having issues at home, that it may require me to take more time off, and that I would not be able to take on additional duties. I was repaid unkindly in one instance when I missed an oral board meeting where I was supposed to participate in pre-hire interviews. I missed the interview, and my boss called me asking where I was at. I was driving one of my children back from a counseling session, and I explained I was dealing with family issues in line with our very recent conversation. He scolded me and told me it was not a good look for someone wanting to be a Captain. I apologized to him while my daughter sat in the back seat.

Later that week, I went to see my Major. I sat with him and was very vague about my day shift position request. I told him that I felt like a *pussy* for even having the conversation, but midnights were having a horrible effect on me, and it was causing problems at home. He was attentive and asked if I would be willing to go to another district if a dayshift position could be accommodated. I declined and told him I did not want to leave the leadership team. In reality, a move to any other district office would be farther from home, causing more travel time and missing more time with my family. My choices were limited to the frying pan or the fire.

My home life and my physical and mental fitness were raging dumpster fires. Despite my administrative duties slipping, I was still highly functional operationally. My persistent sense of failure or falling short of my unreasonable expectations led me to diminish my personal and professional accomplishments.

I finally confided in a sergeant and a corporal, whom I trusted, that I was having trouble sleeping and would need to *bang out* from time to time. This conversation was limited to sleep and none of the other issues. They were incredibly supportive and even called me to ensure I made it home safely. I woke up just before driving under a stopped semi on more than one occasion. I left the sergeant in charge of the platoon so that I could go home and try to sleep before the sun came up, hoping that was the secret. Sleep masks, ocean noise, and blackout curtains weren't working, and I hoped this would. It provided some relief, but it was temporary. This is where my issues began to present themselves at work.

I was in full retreat by this time and had not admitted it. Fear of negative perception, losing my command, or losing my career drove me to press on, hoping to be promoted or sent to the day shift for a reprieve. Promotion was a pipe dream because I knew I was slipping; relief in that form may not come quickly enough. Despite my misplaced priorities and shortfalls, Michelle was always there.

When I left my shift early, I would keep track of my time on a sticky note and back out the time at the end of the pay period. Over time, this practice also went by the wayside, and I left it to memory, hoping that I would recall dates and times over two weeks. I was fully aware there was a cognitive decline, and my memory was foggy at best. This was the second misstep and only added to my problems later. Trying to recall log-off times was difficult, and I did not try to research it myself at the end of the pay period. Over the next few months, this became common practice. Minutes became hours, and they all added up. I was paying such little attention that I even failed to enter overtime that I had worked.

Foreshadowing: A policy memo was issued in September 2016 stating that each employee must complete daily payroll, punch-in, and punch-out for timecards. Before this policy, all payroll was done at a supervisor's discretion, either at the beginning or the end of the pay period. I was aware of this policy.

Despite all my internal issues, there were no outward signs to the platoon or my bosses. Morale and activity were high. I never missed a phone call; I was always available, still actively showing up on calls, and never missed a call I needed to respond to. The sergeant I confided in had known me for over twenty years by this point and knew something was going on, and I was quickly reaching a critical point. He did well managing and filling in where needed. On a particular call, a family had gathered for a birthday when they located the family's patriarch in the greenhouse with a self-inflicted gunshot wound to the head. I responded to the scene, and he was kind enough to brief me in front of the residence. He knew I did not need another ghost or wailing family members.

I was losing what little grip I had on my family life and professional life. They were both tanking, and that led to deeper depression and later increased anxiety and panic. The depression and cognitive distortions led to negative self-beliefs, and I was convinced that I was a piece of shit and Michelle would soon know it. I felt unworthy of love. I believed any conversation I had with Michelle would be the one where she told me as much and that she was leaving me.

I wanted to know what was wrong with me, but I could not ask anyone. One night at work, I went on the Veterans Administration (VA) website and looked at the symptoms of PTS. I could feel my chest tightening as I read the list of symptoms. I had nearly every one of them and had been experiencing them as far back as memory would serve me. I could not get my shirt, armor, and gun belt off quickly enough. I quickly locked my office door and had a panic attack in my office on the floor. Anxiety and panic attacks would visit me regularly, sometimes several times a week, over the next eight months. Being alone during the day and isolated at work helped to keep them hidden from anyone for fear of jeopardizing my career and marriage. I convinced myself I could handle it alone, and this needed to run its course. I needed sleep. I could beat it; I just needed a win.

From March 2019 to November 2019, my platoon experienced a rapid turnover of supervisors. Three sergeants and three different corporals cycled through. Of these transfers, I received one or two sergeants who I believed were less than capable of running one of the squads or overseeing the platoon should the need arise. I felt they lacked decision-making abilities or acumen within patrol operations. I did not choose them, but I was responsible for them.

There were some missed opportunities for communication, such as when they did not brief me on important events while I was on other calls. Two rather critical events required the investigations to be reworked due to a shortfall in their decision-making abilities and lack of patrol experience. There was no impact on either investigation, just some slight embarrassment and the need for follow-up. Although I could claim no blame for their decision-making, I was the platoon commander; the ultimate responsibility to train or relieve them rested with me. Despite several significant successes, these two shortfalls were left glaring. I was in a trough and needed a win, and I needed one quick. The situation was critical and had been for some time.

The Family Academy

In October 2019, the office planned a *family academy*. I was interested in this idea and unsure what it was, but I wanted Michelle and me to attend. We arrived, and another sergeant and I were the only two supervisors in attendance. The rest of the attendees were deputies and their spouses. As it turned out, this academy was about family and resilience.

Presentations about the employee assistance program and our new suicide prevention and resiliency program were given, and a few couples spoke on marriage issues that they had experienced and resources that the office had that they used. Although awareness campaigns and a robust peer support team were already in place, this was the first outward sign that the office supported mental health initiatives. Still, I knew I needed help but stayed silent.

The Break

I understand the act of suicide and understand where some who have died by suicide, attempted, or contemplated may have been in the days and moments leading to their decision. I have been to countless scenes where the elderly, infirm, first responders, veterans, and even children have died by suicide, but despite all my exposure to it, I could never reconcile this as an option for me until now.

One week after the family academy, the wheels finally fell off on October 19, 2019. On shift, I was sitting in my car behind a school. It was about 3 a.m., and I was all alone. Looking out the windshield, I was consumed by hopelessness. For the first time, I considered something I had never contemplated. I thought, *there is a pistol on my hip; I can end it all right now.* I would be free. I noticed my hand on my pistol, and this truly shook me.

The idea shocked me even more when I realized that if I had done it, no one could explain why. As far as I was aware, no one knew I was suffering, no one knew the pain I was in, and I had not asked anyone for help. I contemplated my thoughts for the remainder of the shift and went home.

My Angel

I got home around 6 a.m. and found Michelle awake, sitting in bed. I knew this was never a good sign. I stood at the end of the bed, still in full uniform. She looked like she had been crying. Michelle had no idea what I considered just hours before and would not know about it for many months. She also had no idea that for months, I had convinced myself that I was unworthy of love and that she would leave me at any point. In my mind, this was it. The other foot was about to drop.

Michelle looked at me and asked if I would consider going to marriage counseling with her. I fell to both knees, with hands crossed, as if in a confessional, and pleaded with tears in my eyes. A resounding *yes, anything* to save us. I swore to call the employee assistance line and look for a marriage counselor at the first opportunity. The first appointment I could get was October 31. In the meantime, we continued as if help was on the way. I still had not said anything to Michelle about how I had been feeling or my thoughts of suicide. I tried my best to shake it off; the best I could do was maintain.

Teammates

The following weekend, October 26th, we went to a bar with friends for a few drinks. This was not normal behavior because I wouldn't say I like crowds, especially when they have been drinking. But this was an exception. It was a bar that I had been to on several occasions. This bar was different because it was where we would go after a *trip* when I was at the command. It was this place or a smaller bar on Bay to Bay Blvd. If not a bar, then Uncle Paddy's place. No matter what, there was Guinness, Jamesson, and House of Pain playing. I was comfortable there, and we went with friends.

So, there I was in this bar. I was surrounded by friends, beside the woman I loved more dearly than my next breath. I found myself staring into the glass of Jamesson, neat. I had not even taken my first sip. Despite being surrounded and physically safe, I could not shake feeling alone in a crowded room. It did not make any sense. We sat in the same corner we would sit in when we visited after trips many years ago. Just then, looking into my glass, my thoughts went to my teammates. I took out my phone, took a picture of the glass, and posted it to Instagram. I tagged my teammates and posted *to us and those like us*. I put my phone down on the table and reached for my drink. As I did, my phone came to life. My teammates began commenting and liking the post nearly as quickly as I had posted it. It was almost as if they had been waiting for me. I could not help wondering if they knew how I felt about leaving the command and letting them down.

The Session

On October 31, 2019, we attended our first marriage counseling session. The counselor was very friendly and attentive. I was as open as possible, anticipating that there would be a list of things we needed to do to save our marriage and family. I was tense, but the hour ended, and there was no answer. The counselor told us that she does not counsel couples like us. I thought that signaled the end; I believe I rolled my head backward in response to her statement. She did not mean we were hopeless at all. She told Michelle and me we needed to work on boundaries and communication and offered reading material we could work through together.

The trouble in our relationship was a symptom; I had been numb and emotionally unavailable for years and I needed help. Michelle was patient and had been communicating, but I was deaf to it all. The counselor knew it, and Michelle knew it. I was in the dark on this one.

I was facing the possibility that I could lose my family, knowing I was broken, and yet I was still refusing to ask for help. That was until the counselor turned her attention to me. The counselor asked me directly how my mood was in general.

She asked me if I was high, low, or moderate. Before I could answer, Michelle responded for me. *He's low, and nothing brings him joy.* I tried to deny it with paltry examples of things that brought me joy, and she quickly corrected me, pointing out that the examples I had given were passing amusement and not joy. I did not know what to think of this.

The counselor then asked how I had been sleeping. Michelle quickly responded again. *He doesn't sleep, and he doesn't dream. If he does, it's a nightmare.* She then explained that nearly every night I have been home for the past fifteen years, she has laid awake and watched me as I slept. She told the counselor that I grit my teeth, fight in my sleep, cry in my sleep, and stop breathing just before gasping for air. She said it was heartbreaking to watch me sleep.

I realized that the woman I thought despised me, the man I was, who I had become, had spent her waking moments paying attention to every breath I had taken for at least the past fifteen years. I was so confused. Why are we here? The counselor suggested that I meet with a specialist to address the possibility that I may have PTSD. She suggested the VA and some of her colleagues.

When we left, I was still baffled, and Michelle explained that she did not want me to be mad at her, but this was the only way she knew to get me to a counselor for help. She explained she needed a neutral party to point this out because she did not want me to feel as if she were being critical of me. She saw and experienced every change in me, and despite my best efforts to hide and maintain, she saw it all and still held on. She loved me fiercely and did all she could to comfort and save me. Even to that point, she was afraid to hurt me. Now, Michelle knew my secret, and I was not alone anymore. Later came the realization that I had never been alone. Michelle was and continues to be my hero, shield, and retreat.

Culturally Competent

The information from the family academy and our resiliency program was still fresh. The clinical psychologist who assisted in developing the office's resiliency program was a retired deputy and former soldier. He was not affiliated with the office in any way. I knew him, and I felt safe speaking to him. I reached out immediately. I was able to sit with him in mid-November, and we began my counseling.

Counseling with the Doc differed significantly from the marriage counseling session I had attended with Michelle. First, Michelle was not with me. Second, the marriage counselor was a licensed mental health counselor, not a clinical psychologist. The most crucial difference between this experience and the former was that the Doc had been a soldier and deputy sheriff. He was *culturally competent*. I did not have to explain acronyms or build out the back story for an event. He understood what it meant to wear armor and place yourself in a dangerous position for someone else.

I met with the Doc on several occasions, and at the end of the second session, he explained PTS to me. He laid out the signs and symptoms in greater detail and expressed them clinically. He went further, gave me examples, and connected them with the information from our previous sessions. The Doc explained that per the DSM-5, I met the criteria for PTSD, anxiety, and major depressive disorder. Finally, it had a name. He quickly connected me to a non-profit to assist with paying for the sessions. He was my guide and early advocate, ensuring I met with the VA.

Even though I had been diagnosed with PTS and Michelle and I knew the way forward, there was much more work to be done. This was not the answer but a flag in the ground, a starting point. I was still guarded and did not mention any of the sessions to anyone at work. I increased my conversations with the platoon about mental health. My general demeanor changed because I now knew that what I had been experiencing was not abnormal. I had normal responses to abnormal situations and lots of them. I at least had hope that I could work on my marriage. This experience reinforced the knowledge that speaking with a trained person while you are in crisis, or better before you need them, is much better than trying to self-diagnose and certainly better than self-medicating. I was on the mend, and I hoped for better days ahead.

The Case

There was a way forward for my family. As for my career, or at least as a supervisor, the end was near. On November 19, 2019, my Major called me into his office. There were some concerns about a decision regarding an event in late October after I logged off and went home early. Coincidentally, this was the first time I left one of the newly transferred sergeants in charge of the platoon. A decision was made on a call that would never have been made were I still on duty. To be clear, you can delegate authority but never responsibility. I placed authority in the wrong hands; it was my decision, and ultimately, I was responsible.

The staff reviewed the supervisor's decision, and the only question asked was, *where was Doug?* I was told the question was followed by, and this *would have never happened if Doug had been working.* This search for the answer to their question revealed that I logged off at 0300 hours, the event occurred at 0315 hours, and my payroll said 0600 hours. This discovery was made before I corrected my pre-completed payroll for that pay period.

I explained to my Major that I began filling in payroll at the beginning of the pay period and back out the times for corrections at the end of the pay period. I informed him that I kept notes and approved payroll at the end of the pay cycle. I fully admitted that I knew of the policy and was obviously in violation of the policy.

The Major then asked if I was short on hours. I was surprised and told him I generally kept good notes but left it to memory as time passed. Admitting I was not infallible, and since he asked if I was short on any of my entries, I was queued to the possibility that some of my entries may have been off. He asked if I were to guess, and I could not provide him with an answer. He dismissed me and said that he would report this to the department commander and would be in touch.

I went home and immediately told Michelle what had happened. Later, the Major called me and told me there would be an inquiry since the issue was with payroll. I understood completely and told him I would answer any questions and do any adjustment memos to surrender my accrued time to cover any balances owed.

The notification of an internal inquiry is usually enough to send someone into crisis or cause a marked increase in anxiety. Luckily for me, the severity of my symptoms had been significantly reduced since the first counseling session and my brief work with Doc to that point. When I received the news, I was in a positive, or at least not in a critical state.

I knew the issue was severe, and I fully expected to be

relieved of my platoon and assigned administrative tasks during the inquiry, which was common practice. Contrary to any other supervisor inquiry I had ever heard of, I was left in command of my platoon, and none of my duties changed. Retaining my command and duties indicated that I was still trusted to lead and perform despite my oversight. My Major later confirmed that there was never a question about my ability to perform or lead. Although I expected a punitive outcome, I hoped it would not be fatal to my career and used retaining command to justify this thought.

Let's be clear: I violated a very simple and necessary policy. My lack of discipline here was just symptomatic of the larger issue. The larger issue was that I was knowingly suffering; everything was falling apart, and yet I refused to acknowledge or seek help. I hoped I could handle it alone. *Hope is not a plan.*

Back to Counseling

I continued counseling with the Doc and later with the VA. The Doc made a great point during one of the earlier sessions and noted my negative self-image and self-deprecating thoughts may not have been shared by everyone. He noted that no one is perfect, that I was not Superman, and that I may place my expectations too high. He asked what advice I would give one of my troops if they approached me and reported they had been experiencing the same issues I was; what would I tell him? That was simple. I would tell them to give themselves a break, and we could find the resources together to get them healthier. I felt like an asshole as soon as the words came out of my mouth. It was a statement so simple that it required no thought on my part. The Doc asked why I would give someone else better advice than myself. He told me to give myself a break and pointed out that I may be the only person with this low opinion of myself and should investigate it.

I wanted to start at the beginning. The following day, I started calling some of my former teammates. Outside of Michelle and two other close friends, I felt they would be the only ones to answer me honestly. I called them one by one and was completely surprised. Of those I called, each one told me they had been waiting for this call for years. They each said this is why they told me to get help and get into the VA for all those years. Despite my refusal, they continued to try and convince me to get help, and I would respond by saying things like *I did not rate it* and did not go *down range* with them. They knew how I felt about not deploying with them and that it could only be compounded by the stresses that I must have been under as a law enforcement officer, that it was just as important, if not more important, that I speak to someone about it.

This response was unanimous. They told me that they understood the only reason that I did not go down range was that I was physically unable, I did not have a choice, and I would have certainly gone otherwise. One mate told me that *it was never your pack to carry*. More shockingly, some also knew this was why I did not extend my orders or reenlist in 2007. The Doc was right; I was the only one that thought I was an asshole. I had been seeking vindication or reprieve from a belief no one shared. More than that, I ended a fourteen-and-a-half-year military career on a false perception.

It was now mid-December 2019. I had just turned forty-six. I followed Doc's advice to go to my primary care provider and requested a full blood panel for hormones and cortisol and a sleep study. I met with my primary and brought him up to speed on my issues. After a long and thorough conversation, he prescribed a *beginning* dose of an SSRI and wrote orders for a complete blood panel and a sleep study.

The bloodwork results came back. All the primary organ functions were good to go. My good cholesterol was in the dump; my total testosterone was again low, in the high 180 range. This was not a surprise because I had been on testosterone replacement therapy since my mid-thirties when I began treatment after I encountered the most common problems related to low testosterone. At the time, my number was 168. Though I was higher than my initial levels a decade earlier, my PC started me on a healthier dose and remarked that average numbers are thought to be in the 600 to 800 range. He also said that that's normal based on the average dude sitting on the couch and that my normal may be much higher. He committed to treating the patient and the symptoms, not the lab results. I was diagnosed with hypogonadism and put on testosterone replacement therapy. After trial and error, my PC ran me through a battery of blood work and some subjective questioning about how I had been feeling since starting my TRT. He determined my *normal* level is over 1000. Coincidentally, cortisol was out of balance in my mid-thirties and was still unbalanced at forty-six.

I underwent a sleep study with an *at-home* kit. My sleep study lasted two hours and thirty-eight minutes. That equated to a night's sleep for me at the time. I was diagnosed with obstructive sleep apnea. My primary care physician was amazed I had been functional at all.

As counseling sessions progressed, Doc told me that as I got healthier, other people would see the changes and be drawn to me. They would not know why, and I would not have to say anything. He said that people would want what I had. He was right. Within two weeks of that conversation, seven deputies sought my advice, five of whom did not work for me. This was a significant risk for them to take, and they placed a great deal of trust in me to react appropriately. They were stronger than I had been, and I could not wait to show them the path.

The deputies would come to my office or meet me on patrol. It was always just the two of us, and I listened with genuine interest. I knew where they were and where they were headed. One deputy said he felt like something was pulling him to see me. He sat in my office and cried. He said he felt like a *pussy*, that there was nowhere else for him to turn. I stopped him and asked if he thought I was a pussy? Of course, he said no. So, I told him what I had been going through. What I had gone through. Of course, I only hit the wave tops. I did not need to share everything, but the bits I shared were relatable. As time progressed, I began speaking more regularly about mental fitness and the need to talk about issues and deal with mental health. I wanted to reduce the stigma and fear around the topic as much as possible, but I was not fully invested in being vulnerable.

My family life and work life began to trend upward. The investigation was still ongoing, but I had a path. Understanding that what I was experiencing were normal reactions and adaptations to abnormal events gave me hope, and medication reduced the edge. After being notified about the case in November, I was back on track and winning daily at work. The platoon's morale was high. Barricaded subjects, shootings, jewelry store heists, nothing was out of our reach, and they smashed every obstacle in their way. Even with my newfound relief, the wins, and a treatment plan, I could not shake the burnout.

The End of the Case

By late January, I was still waiting to be interviewed for the inquiry into my payroll. If you have been through an internal affairs investigation, you are all too familiar with the grind—the broad search for information, mountains of transcribed interviews, data, GPS records, etcetera. The scope of the inquiry was not narrowly focused on my payroll records. It did encompass my payroll, of course, but also my GPS and speed for the year, where I ate dinner, how long I ate dinner, and my performance when, on two occasions, sergeants made mistakes. They even interviewed a retiree who gave me a stellar annual evaluation from July 2018 to July 2019. Professional standards detectives also interviewed the two underperforming subordinates whom I had counseled at least once, the sergeant I had confided in, but oddly, did not interview any of the other five high-performing supervisors who reported to me during this time frame.

I was called in for my interview in the late afternoon. Before my interview, I was disarmed and prohibited from using my phone while reviewing the data uncovered during their inquiry. After a couple of hours, I ended my dive into the materials and notified the supervisor that I was ready to be interviewed. I was armed with several pages of notes for my rebuttal.

Although I had my notes, and they would have explained or at least mitigated quite a few of the interviewees' perceptions, they would not change the fact that I disregarded the simple payroll policy. I put away the pad of explanations and counterpoints; I did not need them. I felt they were pointless. I was wrong, and on the outside chance that I argued the point, there was a stack of other allegations like speeding, leaving my assigned area without permission on meal breaks, etcetera. I still had no idea how much time I was short. I am sure it was provided among the materials, but I had yet to go that far in the case file. I was wrong.

I met with the investigators and moved swiftly through their questions. On one occasion, they were mistaken about an event, and I stopped them and corrected them. I said something to the effect of, *let me help you make your case.* My response and the information I gave were certainly not in my favor, and I think the investigators were a bit shocked. No one ever offered incriminating evidence on record in an IA interview.

At the end of the interview, they asked me to read the list of allegations, the corresponding policies, and the potential punitive results for each. The policies are so vague that they offer some room for interpretation. A person looking to minimize their actions or mitigate discipline can go to the letter of the policy and point out that they did not specifically violate the policy. However, someone with character may view the policy's spirit through a lens of the *bigger picture.* Although it was not uncommon for others to do their payroll weekly or at the end of the pay period, I was in violation and was the only one responsible for my actions.

I reasoned that going out of my area for a meal break at 2200 hours, without waking my Captain for permission, was common practice throughout the organization and that I lived less than two miles down a straight road from my district boundary. Still, it did not give me carte blanche to do it. Also, being on meal break for over 45 minutes was not a mortal sin or an uncommon event; I was the platoon commander and was obligated to set the example. Even while pacing speeders for traffic enforcement, speeding was common but was not authorized. I think you get the picture. I admitted I violated each of the allegations and even gave examples of each of the violations.

Their case was a deadlock. The interviewing sergeant, with whom I had a working relationship built on mutual respect, walked me to my car after the interview. He told me he had always admired my character, which was bolstered by my conduct during the interview. He remarked that no one in his time, or even through rumor, had anyone corrected the interviewer and offered incriminating evidence. He told me I had nothing to worry about; *they don't punish people like you.*

I went back to my platoon and finished the remainder of the shift. As a funny side note, I called my Captain and asked if I could leave the district area to go home for meal breaks. He was surprised I asked. He acted as if it were no issue and could not understand why I asked.

For the next few weeks, I continued my duties as if they were business as usual. My sleep was still substandard, but with counseling, I was able to manage the more significant impact of the symptoms of PTS. It was not an easy road, but I was relatively functional, and I was becoming aware of my triggers. Michelle and I were communicating more. My performance at work was back to winning, as it had been a couple of weeks after starting counseling. Substandard supervisors had retired or moved on to other shifts and were no longer a factor. The platoon was stacking win after win.

The Fall From the Peak of Professional Achievement

Nearly five weeks passed with no decision, and late one night, I was pulled aside by someone I had considered a friend and mentor. He informed me there had been discussions about my case, and I needed to consider the worst-case scenario, an outcome I could live with. I still did not know how much time I was short on my payroll and had convinced myself that I would not be terminated. No one outside of those interviewed knew there was even an investigation. There was no impact on the morale or performance of the platoon or the organization. This was not a wanton and willful act with forethought of malice. I had more than enough time in my accruals and did not even claim the overtime I worked. I was honest and owned every action. If not for any of these reasons, I reasoned that I would be spared because I was left in charge of my platoon and had performed brilliantly while under investigation for three and a half months.

The next afternoon, I was called into the Major's office. He had a large binder on his desk and asked me to sit. I sat down and took my pen out of my shirt pocket. He informed me that a decision had been reached, and I was recommended to be demoted to deputy: a three-rank demotion, the first of its kind. I was praying for grace, which, in a way, I received. It may not have been what I hoped for, but it was grace, nonetheless.

Although I was crushed and could not feel my face, I recall trying to ignore the advice from a Captain seated on the couch to my right. I stared at him vacantly as he chirped away with threats. *I would sign it. If you fight it, they will make it worse. They could charge you criminally. They've fired people for less.* I informed him that while I may not be able to choose the punishment, I do choose how I handle it, and it will never be said that I do not accept full responsibility for my actions. I leaned forward and checked the box indicating that I accepted the recommendation, declined a disciplinary review board, and signed.

This punitive action was historic. Although it was revealed

that my actions were not out of malicious intent or forethought and that there were mitigating circumstances, the recommendation was still a demotion. I was crushed and did not say anything. Before being dismissed, I was warned, "Be careful how you tell this story." With that, I was excused. I did not complete the rest of the shift and took the rest of the night off. I needed time to process what this meant and discuss it with Michelle.

It would be another two weeks after I signed off on my demotion that it would be effective. I ran my platoon for the remaining two weeks, hoping the sheriff would commute my sentence. After two weeks, on a Friday, I was informed that I would report to a different district and work for a sergeant on Monday morning at 0600 hours. There was no official notification from the command staff, my Major, or Captain. The receiving district's Captain contacted me. I knew the entire command staff personally and professionally. Still, this was how I was informed that my time as a supervisor, and to a degree, my career, had effectively ended. I shared the news with Michelle and called the receiving district's Major and my new sergeant, both friends. I knew I could have landed in one of a hundred worse scenarios. Though I was grateful for the soft landing they provided and would still be doing the *job*, this was the day I left the profession.

Chapter 22

The Days and Months After

As anyone would imagine, my response to the demotion was heartbreaking. I knew I was responsible for my actions and completely admitted to all culpability before the case began. Although I disagreed with the extreme punishment, I accepted that there would and should be consequences. Still, I could continue to support my family, work toward my pension, and support the organization, albeit in a different capacity, but it would not be the same.

After the case ended, I spoke with two of my closest friends and explained the ordeal. Everything that I had experienced and explained to them my path forward. They were both relieved for several reasons. First, Joel was grateful that I had a plan and was relieved I was human. Thomas was supportive and reminded me, as Joel had, that I was human.

Back to The Road

I did not take any leave; I was starting over, but now, from a point of experience. In retrospect, I should have taken some time off to process the entirety of the ordeal. But, in true fashion, I put on a brave public face and was determined to drive on. I reported for duty on Monday morning and met with my new major, who was happy I was working there. From his vantage point, nothing had changed. My new sergeant, an old friend, assigned me to a field training officer so that I could take my time getting reacquainted with the 500-foot view. Ironically, my newly assigned partner was someone I trained as a field trainer, and he was ecstatic to ride with me. He was very welcoming and did not ask a single question about the case. Still, no one knew why. Of course, there were rumors and speculation, but nothing close to the truth.

Initially, I reported to work with the soldier mindset that I always had: the *I will show you who I am* attitude. I even said I would volunteer as an FTO or assist with emergency management plans should they desire it and when the time was right. Still, I could not shake my perception that I was being viewed as a *broken toy*.

On my second day back on patrol as a deputy, I called the sergeant who had worked for me just 96 hours before. I asked him to gather the platoon in the mall parking lot so that I could address my new position. I felt they deserved to hear the truth from me. I owed it to them, and they deserved it. He happily agreed. I met with the majority of the platoon at 0200 hours.

I explained to them what had transpired over the previous four months and my actions leading to the investigation. I was very clear that the outcome was in response to *my actions*. I told them this was a cautionary tale of waiting too long to ask for help and trying to do it alone. I explained that I had been a hypocrite for advising them to seek help when needed while I was the most in need and refused to get help.

One sergeant strung together a paragraph of profanities

and kicked in the driver's side door of his car. The rest of the platoon was in shock. They had no clue I had been struggling or that there was an investigation. All but the one sergeant who was aware of the case assumed I had been promoted to captain at the last minute. I ended this meeting with hugs and handshakes, then drove back home.

The Whole Truth—Well What They Would Tell Me

A week after my demotion, on a Friday, I was given a DVD with the entire investigation and instructed to sign a form acknowledging that I had ten days to file an appeal with the county commission. I was also informed that although this was my copy of the complete investigation, it was not to be given or released to anyone. Anyone wanting to review it must complete a records request, and a redacted copy would be provided. Although I had no intention of filing an appeal, it was unfortunate that I was given this information on a Friday, day seven of ten allotted days.

I went straight home after receiving the DVD and gave it to Michelle. I had no idea what was on the DVD other than that it was the case. I had not gone through all the materials provided or read the file before signing off on the disciplinary action, and I did not know how much time I was short on payroll. I gave her the DVD and told her to review it at leisure. After several hours, she called me and gave her opinion. Only then was I told how much time was missing: Forty-eight hours and thirty minutes over eight months. Though it would not exonerate me, they did not bother subtracting the overtime I had worked and had not claimed during that period. By their account, $2,387.01 was the price of my career.

This case broke me professionally for several reasons. The first was the severity of the punishment. It was historic, and I felt it was vicious. Second, no command staff member had enough character to call me and have a hard conversation. Third, I had been disavowed and discarded. Frequent calls from peers asking me for advice or mentorship slowed after November 2019 and were halted in March 2020. It would be eight months before any of my former peers or superiors called me or picked up the phone when I called them. Finally, no one within the organization asked me how I was doing or if I was getting the help I needed; this streak is still unbroken as I write these lines four years later.

However, the most significant lesson here has yet to be mentioned because I did not want it to get lost. I was 100% transparent with Michelle during this entire ordeal. She got the unvarnished and unaltered information as I received it—the play-by-play during and even the vicious and disgusting rumors after. Giving her all of the information gave her the power to control what she did with it.

A Professional Pivot

I had been an outstanding trainer, mentor, cop, and leader. I expected the organization to care for me the way I cared for it. This was an unrealistic expectation. But now, I was burnt out and felt abandoned and betrayed. I had been separated from my tribe and my purpose. Even though I could manage any scene or situation, it was clear that I would be relegated to patrol for the remainder of my career. I had to complete 25 years of high-risk service to retire without penalties, and I was only 22 years in. I was left with one of two decisions: I could rededicate myself, stay eight years, and work toward redemption, but ultimately, to what end? Retirement was attractive, but salvation was at least 39 months away. Leaving even a day sooner meant I would be penalized, and my pension would be reduced by 30%.

Complicating matters even more, COVID was in full swing. It was the late spring and summer of 2020, and now I had a body camera on my chest. I was not looking for any opportunity to be questioned. It was clear that keeping a low profile would be in my best interest. During COVID, there was not a lot of proactive police work, primarily situational action and obligatory calls for service. So, this was the perfect opportunity to combine my two options. I rededicated myself to the profession and looked forward to retirement. I modified my work habits. I worked hard when I worked; I was the man they needed when they needed me. I took point, smashed in doors, and generally was the old me, but on my terms—only when I wanted to and only when I was the one for the job.

I informed my supervisors that I would like to be a field trainer and assist with the district-level emergency management plans at a time when they felt it was appropriate. During that time, a friend of mine was tasked with building a new field training course, and he called me asking for the materials I had developed and delivered for years. Although he had not called me in months, I happily sent him everything. I even offered to help him teach it and never heard about it again; I have not heard from him since then. This was the last thing they needed to replace me. My offers to reengage went unfilled for two years before I stopped offering. If you have been around long enough, you know there is the official discipline, and then there is the *double-secret probationary period*, where you get fucked with to see how you react. While I presented my always dependable front for the public, internally, I allowed myself to view my demotion and the denied requests to reengage as a defeat and could not see any route to redemption. They made it clear: I had served my purpose and was no longer needed.

Lacking purpose and relegated to a lower rank, I began feeling sorry for myself. Fully embracing the victim mindset, I gave away my love and passion for the profession and allowed myself to believe I had been betrayed by the institution I had devoted my adult life to. I gave away my joy every time I looked at my uniform. I would become physically ill and suffer anxiety and deep depression on the night before my shifts. This is where I built my house and lived for nineteen months.

The Hits Kept Coming

Moving backward a bit, in February 2021, eleven months after the demotion and my abrupt return to the rank of deputy, I was contacted by the sergeant and asked to come to the district to accept a subpoena. This was a rare event, but it did happen occasionally. I arrived at the district and met with the sergeant and one of our civil process servers. I begrudgingly signed for the subpoena and assumed it was for a civil case where I would be the character witness in a divorce or child custody case. That would have been better.

I opened the subpoena, and it was addressed to me directly. It informed me that the Criminal Justice Standards and Training Commission held a preliminary hearing and decided there was enough evidence to proceed with an administrative hearing for the charge of falsification of official documents, which, if found guilty, would revoke my certifications. They wanted to pull my ticket and I was given a choice. I could elect a hearing and possibly a trial or voluntarily surrender my certifications. Fight or flight? Eleven months after my most significant professional shortfall, I was being tried again for the same thing. Michelle and I both agreed there was no other choice. I had already rolled over and showed my belly to the office. I had to fight and I hired a lawyer that day.

Moving forward, I shared the notice with my chain of command, who then notified the command staff. False outrage from command staff members was followed by promises that I would be taken care of and comments about the unfairness of double jeopardy. Yet, there I was. Luckily, Michelle, as always, was there to help sort the puzzle pieces and research the processes.

My attorney told me there were new members on the disciplinary board, and they vowed to clean up the profession in response to the events of mid-to-late 2020. The board reviewed any cases that were within its purview. My case and more than 1,300 law enforcement officers' cases from around the state filled its growing docket.

My attorney advised me to seek a hearing and accept any plea they may offer. This sage advice cost $2,000.00. I waited patiently over the next nine months, watching hearing after hearing, and there was no mercy. The board had the final say; your only recourse was requesting a trial or appeal.

In September 2021, I returned to my original district with a renewed sense of self. Despite the subpoena months prior, I was happy to be back in a familiar place where my professional value had been established regardless of the title. After brooding for nearly nineteen months, I felt there would be a resurgence, and I would continue improving in all aspects.

Not Without Bad Days: The Happiest Place on Earth

By early fall 2021, I had been managing my symptoms and triggers relatively well. Relative to my typical previous reactions of avoiding or compartmentalizing. Even though I was outspoken about trauma in the responder community, I was still hiding. I was minimizing a lot of my symptoms and issues because I did not trust my organization or that the profession had my best interests in mind. Frankly, I feared the stigma and any further damage to my career. This eased with more time and counseling.

Although I was getting better with time and counseling, some days and situations were managed at a less-than-optimal level. One such occasion happened in October 2021 when the family and I went on a routine long weekend at Disney World.

All had been going well, and we were leaving the Magic Kingdom and going to Epcot. On the way out, my daughter asked to use the restroom, so my wife, son, and I stood on the curb outside of the town hall. I was scanning the crowd and started to get spun up for no reason. I was anxious about something, but there was no stimulus or trigger other than the large crowd.

My face was numb, and my fingers started tingling. I noticed a large family walking toward me. Like every other family, they were smiling and having a great day. Suddenly, all outside noise disappeared, and the crowd surrounding this family seemed to blur. I have no explanation for why, but I was tuned into this family. As they got closer, a cell phone rang. I was close enough to hear the younger woman say hello in a conversational tone. Suddenly, the young woman stopped in her tracks. I saw the lifeless expression on her face. I had seen the look before, and it was as if I were the only person who knew what was coming next. My hands went numb, and my feet got heavy. The girl handed the phone to an older lady in the group, who was still laughing. She took the phone and had a confused look on her face as she said, "Hey." I swear to God, I can still hear her wail as I sit and write this. A soul emptying, "NOOOOOOOOOOOOOO!" She was on her knees and wailing on the ground as her husband ran to her. He grabbed the phone as others tended to her. Confusion and disbelief, the father screamed, "What, no!" I watched this unfold, and I immediately knew that whoever was on the other end of that call had just told her one of her children was dead.

This was the first and only time in my life that I was frozen. I was powerless to help and did not attempt to rush to them. I knew there was nothing anyone could say or do to assuage this pain. This would happen with or without me, and I was disgusted by my reaction.

My field of view suddenly widened, and everyone stood there watching this family in the middle of Main Street. Thank God, one man moved to them. The man was wearing a khaki OD green shirt and hat with a subdued American flag—he was the one they needed at that moment. He took the phone and said they would call back. He helped pick the woman up and usher her off with cast members.

I looked around at the gang of jackals, the fucking heathens gawking at this family, or worse walking by undisturbed as the event unfolded. I was sickened by their reaction and even more so by mine. I turned to Michelle, who was standing next to my 14-year-old son. Our daughter had just walked up and missed the initial part of the event. I stood there like one of the sheep, powerless in front of my wife and son. All I could think about myself was, *You fucking coward!*

Michelle looked at me like I had never seen her look at me. She knew I was done. My cup was too full, and I could not process what had happened. She had an idea of what had happened but was not sure. My son was wide-eyed and frozen. I said it was time to go, and we moved to the exit.

On the walk to the monorail, my children asked what happened, and Michelle said she did not know. Being the sensitive helicopter parent that I am, I said, very matter of fact, that there is only one thing in the world that causes someone to make that noise. I told them that someone told her one of her children was dead. I pressed on and did not even miss my stride. Just when you think you cannot fuck up the dad game even more-BOOM! I was handing out trauma like Oprah used to give away cars.

At the time and in the weeks following, I thought myself a coward for this one action, or lack thereof. If you're unaware, a coward is the C word for those who consider themselves a warrior. With this damaging and underserved self-belief, I dismissed every courageous action I had ever taken. I traded all of it for this ten-second sound bite, a moment of natural human emotion. In my perception, following this event, the past did not matter regardless of the hundreds if not thousands of times I reacted appropriately; I did not act when it counted. I held on to this belief for weeks.

With time and distance to offer perspective, I found that self-deprecating thoughts lead to self-deprecating actions, self-doubt, shame, guilt, anger, and, sooner or later, a wagon full of undeserved imposter syndrome. I was slowly able to process this event and find valuable lessons. First, I am still human and vulnerable to the same emotions as anyone else. At that moment, I was full, and I did not have the emotional capacity to take on another tragedy. Also, I have learned that having positive beliefs about myself and giving myself a break, if not permission to be imperfect, has allowed me to work beyond many of these thoughts and feelings. However, the most important lesson I learned is that response and reaction are very different. If I had paused and used that silence to process what happened and how to explain this, or if I had decided that it needed an explanation, I would not have needlessly exposed my children to further trauma. I learned to use discernment and tact to explain things to my children. I put my newfound knowledge into practice and talked about the event with my kids. I apologized for my behavior when I explained what I thought had happened. They confided in me that it was sad, but they could move past it.

The Suspension

In early November 2021, twenty months after the end of my case and demotion, the state board offered me a plea deal that included a 90-day suspension of my certification, one year of probation to follow the suspension, and completing a prescribed ethics course. This was better than changing careers after twenty-three and a half years and losing forty percent of my pension. In doing the math, I thought about the cost of ninety days without pay, $2k in legal fees, and the loss of $33k a year upon demotion, which was more than anyone should bear professionally, but it was better than the alternative. I adopted the same attitude as before. I did not have the luxury of choosing my punishment, only my response. I accepted the plea as my attorney had advised.

I did not have to wait much longer for a decision. In late November 2021, I was notified that the state board decided to accept my plea and suspended my certification for 90 days, with no pay, followed by a year of probation. In this instance, this was the best I could hope for. The ordeal was distasteful and unfair, but they did not take my ticket. Twenty months earlier, I had been clipped and had just pulled out of the emotional nosedive. On the surface, I appeared to be taking the entire ordeal as a complete Stoic; internally, I had been crushed again.

Unlike the case and demotion, I now had time off to process everything that had happened over the previous two years. I had previously taken ownership of my circumstances as they were largely self-inflicted and could have been mitigated or avoided altogether. I believed I had control over my responses to events and circumstances and could have handled my internal response to the demotion better. There was work to be done. I reframed my situation and took a healthier perspective. I used this 90-day unsponsored hiatus as an opportunity to heal.

In the 28 years of my professional life before this point, I never allowed myself time to process any level of trauma or process the implications of the case and my demotion. My transition from military service post 9/11 back to civilian police work, and years later, my demotion to deputy was literally over a weekend. Forty-eight hours is what I gave myself to switch gears or sort shit out. I had never taken a long enough break to realize how much stress I was under. I had become accustomed to the grind. Now I had the time. I quickly learned that I was free from the Sunday gloom—the nausea and anxiety I had experienced for the previous two and a half years. I could now see this picture fully as I was no longer in it.

I did some deep work on myself and kept busy. I used the next 90 days to train for and run a marathon, double up on my master's classes, and learn to be present for my family. Running and reading were easy, but being present was foreign to me and my family. It required work, but I loved it. I quickly adapted to my role as husband, dad, and Doug.

Training, studying, and being a present husband and dad were awesome. A friend I had kept in touch with during this time called to check in on me, and it turned into a 45-minute conversation about my kids and what they have been up to. Eighty days before this call, the conversation would have been summed up with *the kids are good*. I had a wonderful time with my family and accomplished a lot of deep work on myself—the suspension's positive effect on my physical and mental fitness was glaring. This was a gift.

I reminded myself that playing the victim or the victim mindset, even internally, permits you to dismiss responsibility for the events in your life. Victimhood is the easy route, and I was no victim. Regardless of the consequences, I owned every bit of my part in my troubles. I had not been run off and was the only one who thought I was broken. I vowed to be more mindful about how I spoke to myself.

Through it all, no matter how bad it got, even after suicidal ideations and a loose plan, I still did not take myself out of the fight. I continued to bash my head into a wall figuratively. Ultimately, it was Michelle's request to go to counseling to seek help that pulled me from the bottom. As distasteful as this entire string of events was, they were necessary. This had to happen as it did. In truth, the organization merely changed what was on my shirt and removed themselves from my list of distractions. When it was all done, I would be stronger than before.

A noteworthy addition to this section is that this person, referenced above, was the only person to call and check on me during my 90-day hiatus. Neither my *closest friends* nor the command staff, who were outraged that I was being subjected to this treatment, picked up the phone.

A New Perspective

Ninety days later, my penance was paid in full. When I returned to work, there was an opening at the district desk. The desk deputy position was typically reserved for the old-timers transitioning to retirement or younger troops looking to hide. Regardless of which class you fell into, the position did not carry a high level of regard. The position consisted of administrative tasks around the district and was a catch-all for any walk-ins or deputies needing assistance. Additional benefits came with the position: twelve hours less driving daily, a highly reduced likelihood of controversy or complaints, the benefit of air conditioning, and a roof.

I was offered the position and struggled with the idea for a bit. I considered the perception of others if I had made this move. What would they say? Burnt out, salty, and on a desk. *Look where all the hard work got him: an old guy nobody listened to. He used to be dangerous, the best deputy in the entire district, and is now relegated to what used to be.* My ego was trying to dissuade me. I made some phone calls and spoke with Michelle about the opportunity. The feedback was unanimous, and I decided the smart move was risk reduction and the beginning of a long off-ramp to retirement.

I did not have to wait for long for the opinions of others to reach back to me. In the first couple of weeks, there were occasions when deputies from other divisions came in and shook their heads in disbelief. Some even said they heard I was working at the desk and had to see it themselves. "I never thought Doug White would be at a desk." I disregarded what others' perceptions may have been and reframed my situation. This allowed me to focus on the positive aspects of the assignment. I quickly realized that I was now in a central place, available to all deputies, detectives, and supervisors, and I had direct access to the district command staff. I was the first person everyone met when they walked into work each morning, and I took full advantage of daily opportunities to train and mentor younger deputies and supervisors.

The bosses were happy when I took over the desk assignment. I functioned with the professional knowledge of a lieutenant, which led to supervisors, even my major, asking me for input on personnel and professional issues. I brought stability and professional knowledge to the position. There were no operational or professional situations for which I was not suited. I was low-maintenance and completely self-sufficient. Though in a much different capacity, I had a professional purpose again. I finished my last year as a desk deputy.

Chapter 23

Transitioning

I knew my time in law enforcement had a shelf life, and it was rapidly approaching. I had driven hard for more than twenty-seven years, and although I had not driven as hard for the last three years, I was still in the fight. I did not know how to stop and felt I needed to have something lined up the next day after retirement. Not only was this feeling attributable to my drive, but I was also asked what I would do next. I was asked this question repeatedly, and it became a million-dollar question. I had no answer. I had no idea what I wanted to be after retirement. I had been a sledgehammer for nearly thirty years and needed to sharpen my scalpel skills. I made the mistake of trying to figure this out before I retired, and the day was approaching quickly. In haste, I landed on several ideas, but nothing set me on fire.

    I obtained a master's degree in criminal justice and homeland security to teach undergrad, and I had been accepted into a doctoral program for adult education. After I met the qualifications to teach undergraduate-level courses, I prepared a lesson plan and interviewed for a college. I enjoyed the experience but realized it did not set me on fire. I walked away from the table during salary negotiations, and that was okay. I saved myself another four years of education and a ton of money not pursuing the EdD.

I started reading books and listening to podcasts about transitioning to a new career, pivoting after fifty, and similar topics. I also asked people I knew who had retired or transitioned from the military or first responder communities what advice they would offer. I learned several things from veteran and first responder authors and podcasters who published or spoke about their experiences in these spaces, which were fantastic resources. Their first recommendation was to take time off, if possible, without causing financial harm to yourself or your family. This advice made perfect sense, and I abandoned the idea of transitioning to a new career over a weekend.

Setting up for a smooth transition takes forethought and planning at least one year from your retirement date. Unfortunately, I was within weeks of retirement when I learned this information. I was fortunate enough to be in a position where I had a pension and could take time off after I retired, which gave me breathing room and reduced quite a bit of stress. I also found that answering "nothing" to the million-dollar question was quite the flex.

In the weeks leading up to retirement, I built the foundational elements recommended by the authors and podcasters I had been filling my time with. Networking and a resume were the crucial bedrock on which my next chapter would be built.

Creating a LinkedIn account well ahead of your transition is essential. LinkedIn is a platform for professionals. Start building connections and relationships outside of your current circle. Aim for people in the circles you would like to be involved in. Beware, law enforcement officers are generally straightforward and to the point. Over time, we generally become suspicious of everyone, if not outright hate people, and may find networking complicated as I did. In my case, I was turned off immediately when I began meeting people who showed interest in me only to reach out with an *ask* for me to either make an introduction to people in my network or purchase their leadership and success course on one of their social media platforms. Once I did, I didn't hear from them again. Expect this and be ready with a response when someone approaches you. I found these interactions distasteful and disingenuous, but unfortunately, the business world is transactional, and this is just a part of it.

A resume is essential if you are looking to transition into another career. The hardest part was translating any military or first responder jargon into a language the business world could understand. This takes time. I also learned that each resume should be tailored to the specific position you are applying for. This is not a one-size-fits-most project. Focus on your soft skills if your hard skills are not adaptable. For example, focus on your decisiveness and adaptability, learning ability, emotional intelligence, leadership skills, and the ability to communicate effectively. Being on time for work is not a skill.

The foundational items were in place, and retirement was imminent. It was time to start fresh. I had to consider what I wanted to be, look ahead five to ten years, and decide what I wanted our lives to look like. The questions I started with were: What was my purpose? Where was my mission? What did I need to learn, and from whom or where would I learn it? How would I measure success? How would I know when I reached it? Finding these answers took work. It took critical self-reflection, a lot of reading, journaling, and time. This is not an overnight process and is ongoing nine months after retiring.

The Last Day

July 13, 2023, was my 25th anniversary and my last day at the office. I had to turn in all my gear, and there was a list of things I *owed* the office, and everything the office had issued to me was packed up the night before. As usual, I awoke early, put on my utility uniform, and Michelle performed the ritual of walking me to my truck for the last time. After a last morning kiss, I was off.

My first stop of the day was the range. The range is situated on the county's south end, and I lived on the far north. The drive would take just over an hour at *cop speed*. I was no stranger to this trip to the south county. I cannot estimate the number of trips over the past 25 years. At the beginning of my career, I would visit the range at least one day a week to work on firearms proficiency. As you can imagine, I was assigned to training and was also a firearms instructor for many years, which brought me to range quite a bit. I was a bomb technician for over six years, and we did most of our training and demo at the range. I was alone, just like always, but this trip was different. This would be my last trip to the range. This was the last time I would need to drive this far for anything foreseeable. It occurred to me that the places I would visit during the day would all be my last.

I arrived at the range and went in through the instructor's entrance. I met the range corporal and sergeant with whom I had worked. The meeting was cordial but regimented. All the T's crossed and such. With handshakes, hugs, and well wishes, I was off to the next stop. As I drove away, I felt as if I no longer belonged. A place where I have spent thousands of hours baking in the sun honing my craft or training others, a place where I was familiar with every square yard, now felt foreign to me. I felt like I was leaving someone else's home after an obligatory visit, and they had been waiting for me to leave. I did not belong.

The next spot was supply. I walked in and did not see a familiar face. They looked at me like I was lost and had to explain that I was retiring and needed to turn in my equipment. The entire interaction was, again, regimented and transactional. They just went down the checklist, placing a tick mark next to the item numbers as I unloaded my box.

I handed in my stars and my credential wallet. The friendly clerk smiled and told me to wait; she would get me a new credential wallet for my retired credentials. I thought that was nice, but I never carried my credential wallet in my back pocket like some old-timers, so the one I turned in was perfectly fine. When she returned, she handed me a credential wallet that someone else had turned in previously. I looked at it, and all I could think about was the $600+ million budget and the asinine amount of money wasted on laptop cover decals, and that after twenty-five years, they could not even give me a new $20 wallet or let me keep the one I already had. I was so dumbfounded that I did not consider asking for a new credential wallet. I just wanted to leave. I left there and could not wait to finish the entire ordeal. My visit to the radio shop, evidence, human resources, and benefits were identical. They were transactional, almost as if they had somewhere else to be.

My last stop was Benefits, located on the other side of the large compound across a busy street. No longer having a car, I had to walk a quarter mile and cross the street for my last meeting. With a backpack in hand, I walked through the parking lot. On this short journey, I passed two patrol districts and three divisions clustered together on the sprawling property, then across the street to get to the benefits section. I felt like a dick; it was a walk of shame.

This would be the worst experience of my day. When I finished with benefits, the clerk walked to her office door and pointed to the lobby door. I walked alone to the lobby, the door closed behind me, and that was it. An entire organization open to me five minutes prior was now a secret club—one for which I no longer had a password.

I requested someone accompany me while I turned in all my gear, but we were too short-staffed. I had to call a supervisor to pick me up when I thought I would be done. I texted the sergeant before I got to Benefits to let him know I would be done in roughly twenty minutes. He said he was across the street and would be there when he was done, and it should only be a few minutes. When I was done, I texted the sergeant, and he said he would be right over. I waited on the curb in front of the benefits section, holding a backpack containing what was left of my career, for forty minutes waiting on him. He was on the phone with his brother-in-law when he finally picked me up. After his twenty-five-minute conversation, he hung up and offered some small talk. Even though I had known this sergeant for twenty years and at one point he even worked for me, I felt like I was being Uber'd home by a stranger. Fair enough, I was no longer a member of his tribe.

The entire day left me empty. I did not want a parade but at least someone to acknowledge my twenty-five years of service. I felt like I had dedicated the best years of my adult life and had been rewarded with a used credential case. It became clear that my contributions to the organization ended the day I walked out the door. All the prestige from the position or title bestowed upon me by the organization was left at the door. After all, it was only borrowed anyway.

I got home and settled in for about an hour before I left for the district. Michelle, the district's administrative staff, and my lieutenant coordinated a small gathering for me around midafternoon. Initially, I did not want a *cake party* and preferred to fade away, but they would not hear of it. In my experience, long-serving supervisors were the only retirees who rate a command staff appearance. Although I ascended to the rank of lieutenant, and despite my end-of-career shortfall, I had worked with and directly for most of the staff, not one came to my cake party. Even on my last day, it was made abundantly clear that I had been uninvited to sit at the big kids' table, discredited, disavowed, and now dismissed. One major, who was a friend and whose character rose above the others, attended. The room, however, was full of deputies, detectives, and supervisors I had worked with over the years.

My lieutenant and platoon presented me with a framed photo of me taken during my bomb team days—a moto pic from my youth. The mat around the photo was inscribed with heartfelt and personal sentiments by those who had the opportunity to sign it. Despite retiring as a deputy, most messages began with my former call sign, 3L3 or Lt., or more personally, Doug. As I read the messages, they did not mention my shortcomings; they only referenced the man they knew, my character, leadership, and my impact on them. No one in attendance saw me the way I saw myself: failure, breaking, or broken. To them, I had always been a meat-eating, tooth-chipping enforcer. In their eyes, the only thing the office had changed was my collar brass. Though not infallible, my tireless dedication drove me to be the best I could be; I set the standard, served the profession faithfully, and protected those who could not protect themselves. I left with my character intact; my purpose had been fulfilled. I rated, and I mattered.

The following weekend, I had a proper retirement party and invited some people who had impacted me the most during my career. Ironically, no one from the command staff was invited. There was not a single junior varsity-level person there. They were all highly accomplished, brilliant, Samurai-dangerous warrior poets and had more than their fair share of stories of our adventures together. I was doing my best to speak with everyone and soak in the gravity of this gathering. With Michelle by my side, I stood before them and looked across the room. Most of the group was with their spouses. As I learned, they knew that no one got through it alone.

What Do I Do With My Shadow?

Over the last thirty years, I changed into this persona: driven by purpose and ego, overinvested in an idea, and fed by the perceptions of others that were carefully constructed around me; I gave life to stories that were retold and turned into local legends. I was the shaved head enforcer that scared the scary—the bump in the night and the man that could deescalate with a silent presence and commanding posture. A look, a tone, or even a simple grin gave life to phrases often repeated: *Didn't you get them memo? That's Doug White, motherfucker!* At the end of thirty years, having been this *thing* for so long, one day, I woke up and was no longer this *thing*. No tribe, no next mission, or larger purpose. What am I now?

This question and others became central to my thoughts. I fell into a deep depression, and hopelessness crept back in. For weeks after retirement, I was plagued with suicidal ideations. I reached a point where I believed the only benefit of continuing to breathe was so that my family would continue receiving my pension. I believed that money was the only contribution I could make, and to do that, I would need to be on the grassy side of dirt. Finally, I reminded myself that we all need help; we only need to ask. I sat down with Michelle and explained everything. For me, just saying it out loud seemed to make it better.

Now, with clarity and through a realistic perception of reality, I began to work on finding the answers. I circled back to that moment on Fire Watch thirty years earlier. Nineteen-year-old me could not fathom the journey that lay ahead. I was the man I needed to be to fulfill the roles along my path. My monster and shadow kept me alive. They were necessary to steel my nerves, react with violence and aggression when necessary, and empathize to comfort should the need arise. I was friends with my monster; we were mates, and I could control it, but I no longer needed it lurking around the corner. However, we will remain close, and I can quickly call on him when or if he is needed. As the Chinese proverb tells us, it is better to be a warrior in a garden than a gardener in a war.

What advice would I give if I could visit nineteen-year-old me that morning in the mirror? With the benefit of thirty years of experience, I would say you will be the man you must become to survive what lies on your path. Be cautious, balance this persona with your character, and ensure the persona exists only when necessary. Prioritize—you will be a father and a husband; those roles are, first and foremost, the health and stability of your family will be the measure of your success.

So, what am I now? The answer is now clear to me. I am a father and a husband who works daily to be the best version of myself by combining faith, family, and fitness.

Chapter 24

What Can Be Done?

My former and many other organizations have a peer support team and an employee assistance program (EAP). From my vantage point and the concerns voiced to me, I understand why people hesitate to use these services. First responders generally do not walk around freely talking about our emotions and what we do to address our mental fitness. Apprehension of being vulnerable and the perceived stigma attached to less-than-optimal mental fitness are viewed as career-enders. Internal peer support or an EAP that the organization provides brings confidentiality issues. Maybe someone slips and mentions your issues, or EAP is provided by insurance, who may report usage to the organization. These are all valid concerns, and individual decisions must be made. I used EAP for my children's teen angst issues, and I sought marriage counseling. These seem innocuous enough not to raise a red flag at work.

I have heard suggestions for forgetting about the job and everyone else's thoughts, walking away, and doing something else. I agree with the sentiment, but to some, there is a perception that this job is the only thing you feel you can do; it may have been a childhood dream, or more simply than that, it pays the bills and supports your family.

Some may feel that being vulnerable and asking for help indicates that you cannot handle the rigors of the job, and by asking for help, you place your job in jeopardy. These are the things we tell ourselves. I tried to convince myself that it would get better when I got to the day shift and that it would get better when I was promoted to the next position. This denial or avoidance puts us in the position to continue drinking the poison that has been making us sick. The change starts with you.

What Can Leadership Do?

As a young law enforcement supervisor, I was told that the burden of leadership is having the moral courage to do the right thing. The speaker continued by saying that it is a burden and a privilege. You have earned the privilege to be in a position where you are required to uphold the tenets of the profession and drive forward a culture of service.

Leadership courses and books agree that organizational culture begins at the top. The chief executive sets and communicates the culture, and subordinate leaders ensure it is communicated, demonstrated, and fostered. The adage, *a fish stinks from the head*, holds here.

Organizational leadership must ensure that employees feel safe and valued. A culture viewed as one that *eats its own* will likely never normalize post-traumatic stress injuries or experience the complete dedication of its personnel. Creating a safe work environment where people feel valued, building a culture of asking for help, and rallying around those who seek it instead of alienating them may lead more employees to use the internal programs offered instead of staying hidden. Normalizing the symptoms of PTS and characterizing them as injuries or admitting that these are adaptations and are normal in the context of our work is critical.

Recruit, hire, retain, and promote personnel with strong moral character and the personal attributes found in good leaders, such as emotional intelligence, empathy, decisiveness, critical thinking, and integrity. Train all levels of leadership to recognize the signs and symptoms of burnout, post-traumatic stress, depression, etcetera.

The employee and the organization would be well served if frequent conversations about PTS and normalizing the effects one may experience throughout one's career occurred regularly. This *normalization* should begin in the academy. Frontloading this information allows employees to recognize their potential need for assistance before becoming critical. Being well-informed on the front end also allows employees to make more informed decisions about their future in the profession.

Leadership should take a broader view of personnel performance by searching for cause and effect and working to identify or treat the root of the behavior. For example, I began my military career at nineteen and civilian law enforcement at twenty-four. Assume that each state requires a candidate to be at least twenty-one years old to be hired. They may be twenty-two when they complete training and are working in a solo capacity. A twenty-, twenty-five-, or thirty-year career spans arguably the most critical part of someone's life. Marriage, purchasing a house, birth of children, divorce, loss of spouse, children leaving the house, death of parents, and the list goes on. Circumstances impact the lives of your personnel in ways other than what they are experiencing at work. If the troop is sharp and on top of their game and shows signs of poor performance or a change in demeanor, stop for a moment before swinging the axe and explore what may be happening in their lives that could be responsible for a change.

Leadership should ensure or at least endeavor to measure reprimands and impose punitive discipline fairly and equitably, seeking to add value for the organization and balancing that with the future and well-being of the employee. More simply, ensuring the punishment fits the infraction. Swinging the axe and responding harshly to their behavior during a crisis with disciplinary action fails to address the possible underlying issues. This can be seen as an institutional betrayal that is harder to recover from. This is a lose-lose proposition with second and third-order effects. You are failing your troops and the organization.

Chapter 25

Growth

I did not devise this path to growth on my own. The information that guided me has been borrowed from a dozen books, dozens of podcasts, and articles written by experts in their fields on leadership, transition, PTS, sleep hygiene, physical fitness, mental fitness, nutrition, and mindfulness.

Of the more notable resources were the Camaraderie Foundation, Dr. *Jordan Peterson, Jocko Willink, Mike Sarraille-Everyday Warrior, Cody Alford, Ryan Holiday, Shawn Ryan-Vigilance Elite, Dr. Gabrielle Lyon, Dr. Kirk Parsley, Herb Thomspon, Dr. Dan Pronk, Dr. Phil Bacquie, Jason Palamara, Barbara Rubel, Karl Monger, Nick Koumolatsos, Dr. Chris Frueh, Andy Stumpf-Cleared Hot, Atlas Aultman, Nick Lavery, Dr. Medina Baumgart, Dr. Kevin Gilmartin,* and the list goes on. This is only the beginning of my journey.

Find a Purpose and Mission

For over thirty years, I had a mission, and, in most cases, I was overcommitted and consumed. My retirement marks the first opportunity in my adult life where I am in complete control of my days and where I control to whom I dedicate my time and efforts. I believed I needed a new job or project lined up the week after I retired. I was only forty-nine when I retired and had plenty of work left. I did not know what I wanted to do; I just knew what I did not want to do.

I did not want to work in an environment where personnel are treated as expendable or disposable or where fear of the organization is greater than the dangers of the job itself. I wanted to be in an environment of trust, where everyone is valued and free to contribute. I found this environment inside my home with my family. My new mission is to be the best version of myself for my family and future. If, one day, that leads to clarity and revelation of my greater global purpose through vocation, then so be it. But for now, I am building myself. I am present for my family.

As the months passed, I felt strongly that I wanted to serve my community and advocate for the veteran and first responder communities from a platform of recovery and growth. Six months into retirement, I found a non-profit aligned with this mission. I carefully set clear boundaries and expectations and communicated them with Michelle. Together, we decided to support the charity. When my children are at school and my wife is at work, I fill my time with volunteering for a veteran's service non-profit committed to bringing veterans out of isolation using humor and camaraderie to prevent veteran suicide.

As I continued writing this book, I found that my family and this project consumed most of my time. This was as it should have been and aligned with my boundaries. Focusing my efforts on building a presence for this service organization took little time or effort, but it was enough to pull my focus on completing my manuscript.

Completing this work was critical, and it needed to be published. I found my purpose during this process. All my experiences, owning my journey, and everything tucked in my shadow were now in the light. I found power in vulnerability and honesty. Owning my shit and being bold enough to share the story with anyone who will listen, and from any stage, became a superpower. I am convinced I am still here because this is what I am supposed to be doing, speaking to you through these pages. I am using my voice to drive positive change, break the stigmas, and show Alphas that there is power in using your voice.

Tribe

Invest in your familial relationships. Shore those up by being intentional and present. Communicate and be receptive to your family members' emotions. Evaluate and then do the work. The tribe starts here!

Along with family, I knew I needed to build a network outside my previous circle. I did not necessarily need a network of businesspeople but a network of moral people who had the attributes I wanted to emulate. I wanted a group of men who were present only because they wanted one another to be successful, not in competition, but enabling. Men, who, by their actions and example, I could count on to keep me driving forward and hold me accountable on this journey. Men who I knew to be good family men, honest, and hardworking.

I did not have to go far, and I did not need an entire tribe. I stopped posting to social media and watching daily news. I curated my influences and concentrated on reading for enrichment and seeking men in positions or stages of their lives that I wanted to work toward. I found this through long-distance mentorship through articles, books, or podcasts and meeting in person with select men. I recommend anyone on this path connect with inspiring and uplifting people.

Body, Mind, and Spirit-Spiritual Fitness

I am no expert in this arena, but I know that believing in a power larger than myself is paramount. I am a spiritual person, and I believe in the Divine workings of God. I was raised Christian and attended a Methodist church, and I had a good sense of right, wrong, and morality. Throughout my career, I found myself coming back to the church looking for something good in the world. I was looking for good people and faith in humanity, the *chicken soup for the soul moments,* and less about my relationship with Jesus Christ.

This information was not something that struck me daily and likely should have. I was aware of the Divine presence, but I was lost. I recommend that anyone looking for grounding or answers to their own issues seek help from something greater than themselves, whatever that may be. There are instances where I should have and could have been killed, gravely injured, or simply lost forever, and simply was not. I have no worldly reason for why I was spared, so I must give way to grace. Simply speaking, on many occasions, I was spared by grace alone.

The reason for my salvation became clear during a conversation with Michelle recently. I shared with her that in my lowest, when I was hopeless, sitting in my patrol car in the vacant parking lot, hand on my pistol, and contemplating ending my life, I could not see God. For years, I could not see or hear God. I was lost. I confessed this to her with tears in my eyes. By this point, Michelle was crying, too. Without thought or pause, she asked me, had I considered that I did not have to see or hear God because someone had been praying for my safety for years? Her question landed squarely. She told me she had been up all night before I got home on the morning of October 19th. She was at her end and had been for some time. She was trying to find the resolve to guide me toward help or find the strength to leave me to my own devices. Her love for me and us was too great for the latter. Then, when I walked in and stood at the foot of our bed, I dropped to my knees, and her prayers had all at once been answered. Without Michelle and faith, there is no *happily ever after* to this story.

Physical Fitness

I have some recommendations based on the lessons I have learned. This is not the way, just a way. Physical fitness is linked to mental fitness. Despite the injuries, aches, and pains that come with military service, first responder duties, or simply the infirmities of age, you must remain active. I began training for triathlons as a great way to reduce my stress, stay fit, and find an outlet for my competitive nature. Were it not for physical activity, I would have burnt out years prior, in a time when I was less inclined to listen to reason or seek help.

After medical approval, find a fitness program you enjoy and do it consistently. Physical activity reduces stress, burns fat, builds lean muscle, and regulates hormones like cortisol and testosterone. If nothing else, it is a reason to get out of bed and stretch. Changing your body composition may be enough to change your attitude.

Mental Fitness

Physical fitness and activity, eating healthy whole foods, journaling, breathing exercises, practicing gratitude, and mindfulness have all been effective options. Still, they only delayed the inevitable burnout or bottoming out without culturally competent counseling or therapy. No one gets through alone. Get professional assistance before you are in crisis.

With proper care and attention, PTS injuries are manageable and treatable, and there is a way to win. The goal is to experience post-traumatic growth, to be better and more complete than before because of the experiences. This aligns with Dr. Jordan Peterson's theory, which explains that embracing and taming the shadow described by Dr. Jung, or Peterson's monster, makes you virtuous, a complete person, and moves you toward individuation. This is a daily journey.

My mental fitness journey began with a culturally competent counselor. Later, when I entered the VA system, I found that the providers I had were not veterans, had never served, and were largely clueless about experiences in the veteran or first responder's life. Their response was medication and lots of it. Medication may be part of your treatment plan. You have the right to question, research, and say no if you are uncomfortable with the suggested medications and dosages. You also have the right to take ownership of your care.

Hormone Regulation

For years, I have experienced all of the symptoms associated with low testosterone or hormonal dysfunction. I mentioned that my testosterone level was in the high 100s when I had it checked by my primary physician in my mid-thirties. This was years before seeing him for depression and still years before I sought culturally competent counseling. I would recommend visiting your primary care physician or an endocrinologist. Have a full panel of blood work conducted. I found that regulating cortisol and hormone levels through hormone replacement therapy has had a positive effect on some of my symptoms like depression, fatigue, sex drive, focus, etcetera.

Sleep Hygiene

In 2019, my primary physician ordered a sleep study based on my reported symptoms. As a side note, I had been experiencing the symptoms for the better part of fifteen years before I spoke up. I was experiencing excessive daytime sleepiness, loud snoring, and stopped breathing during sleep. Sometimes, I wake up during the night or day gasping or choking. On occasion, I would wake up with a dry mouth or sore throat, morning headaches, trouble focusing during the day, or mood changes like depression or anger. I learned that sleep apnea leads to several risk factors, and I could reduce it with a mouthpiece specifically for sleep apnea and practicing good sleep hygiene.

Exposure to Toxins or Traumatic Brain Injury

As part of my VA health care system enrollment, I was screened for the PACT Act, Burn Pit Registry, and Traumatic Brain Injury (TBI). TBI may be an overlooked key to the severity of other issues, such as neurological issues, cognition, anger, balance, etcetera.

The TBI screening was a battery of questions asked over

the phone. They ask about any concussions, loss of consciousness, exposure to blast overpressure, significant blows to the head, or firing heavy weapons. Initially, I dismissed all of these because I did not deploy in combat, was never blown up, and did not believe I had any significant exposure. Over thirty years, I have fired my share of rounds and have left long days of shooting training with headaches and nausea; explosions and heavy weapons were a requirement for air base defense missions while I was in the Air Force, and one had to stay familiar with and proficient in their use. I know there was no impact there due to the infrequency of the training.

In my responder role, I have also had my fair share of head-snapping jolts from car crashes, open-field tackles on bad guys, or time in a Redman suit, but I never lost consciousness, as I can recall. My most significant concern came from my time on the bomb squad. Along with being a bomb technician, I was also trained to be a breacher. Overpressure from demolition, counter charges, energetic disruptions, and breaching was a full-body experience. Although there are set minimum safe distances for demolitions and breaches, with or without a shield, I have been close enough that we have had to clean bits of breacher tape off the front of an entry shield and blast blanket or bits of door frame stuck to our helmets or armor. I have left long training days with a splitting headache, nausea, flu-like symptoms, etc. Fortunately, they went away after resting and taking Ibuprofen. Screening may rule out TBI or provide a starting point for your physician.

Moderation and Abstaining

One of the subjects that kept coming up in the reading and podcasts was self-medicating, indulging in destructive activities, or seeking cheap and quick dopamine dumps. They all warned to be conscious and try to avoid overconsumption of alcohol or other medications. Alcohol does not help sleep; in fact, alcohol destroys quality sleep and is a net zero gain. There is no benefit to it. Be aware or try and recognize risk-taking behaviors, compulsive or avoidance behavior like excessive time playing video games, overeating, gambling, and porn. All of these things detract from the healing process. I aim to be the best version of myself and work to that end each day. I concentrate on the three pillars: mind, body, and spirit.

Growth and Beyond

I have found that the path to success or happiness is not linear. There will be bad days. My path has led me in an arc, through switchbacks, and even over a cliff. I can now objectively reflect on my professional journey over the past thirty years and know that my accomplishments, being a teammate, a bomb tech, a teacher, and a leader, are the bona fides of a successful professional life. I am proud of my service and experiences.

I viewed my service to our profession as a worthy cause that deserved and demanded the best of me, and to a fault, I was all in. Opportunities to slow down or ask for help were within my control, and I could have done more to reduce my decisions' impact on me and my family. With the wisdom that comes with time, I would make different personal decisions to mitigate the effects or avoid their impact altogether.

Given the opportunity, I would do it all over again, incorporating the knowledge that my contributions to my family are generational and will continue long after I am gone. The most important titles or roles I will have or fulfill are those of a husband to a loving and dedicated wife and a father to two wonderful children. Restoring my standing in these roles, working to become the best version of myself, and serving my family are my purpose and legacy. Through grace, love, vulnerability, honest communication, and hard work, I have been given a second chance—an opportunity to tell this story.

About Doug White

Doug White's career spans over 30 years of distinguished service to his country and community. He served in the Air Force from 1993 to 2007 as a Security Forces specialist and later dedicated 25 years as a deputy sheriff with a major law enforcement agency in west-central Florida. His roles included patrolman, field training officer, domestic violence and child abuse investigator, advanced training instructor, and certified bomb technician. Doug's leadership positions ranged from supervising patrol services squads and the canine section to commanding the Special Incident Management Section and environmental crimes unit and as a patrol platoon commander after rising to the rank of lieutenant.

Doug's military career began as a security specialist and law enforcement patrolman in the United States Air Force. He continued with the Individual Mobilization Augmentee (IMA) program, serving with the 919th Special Operations Wing and then Headquarters United States Special Operations Command (USSOCOM) for nearly a decade. Following the events of 9/11, Doug voluntarily returned to active duty for 37 months in support of Operation Enduring Freedom and Operation Iraqi Freedom. As a founding member of the Protective Services Detachment, Doug served through the tenures of General Peter Schoomaker and Admiral Eric Olson.

Personal Journey and Mission:

Doug's journey through the shadows led him to the peak of professional achievement and hopelessness and to a vacant parking lot with his hand on a pistol. He has navigated significant challenges with post-traumatic stress (PTS) and the host of physiological and psychological injuries that accompany it. Through grit, Grace, and vulnerability, he has transformed his struggles into a powerful narrative of resilience and growth. His journey from battling PTS to achieving personal growth underscores his commitment to breaking the silence and stigma around mental fitness and injuries experienced in the veteran and responder communities and their families. Doug's story highlights the strength found in sharing one's story and embracing vulnerability as a pathway to healing.

Current Work and Mission with Tell This Story LLC:

As an author and speaker, Doug White is dedicated to empowering veterans, first responders, and their families. Through Tell This Story LLC, his mission is to support individuals in finding their voice and power through storytelling and overcoming the silence surrounding PTS and mental fitness.

Doug can be found on IG at @tell_this_story and on LinkedIn at https://www.linkedin.com/in/doug-white-le2biz/ or by email at info@DougWhiteOfficial.com

Notes

Introduction

1. Jung, C. G. (1968). *The Archetypes and the Collective Unconscious.* Princeton University Press.
2. Jung, C. G. (1968). *The Archetypes and the Collective Unconscious.* Princeton University Press.
3. Jung, C. G. (1981). *Aion: Researches into the Phenomenology of the Self.* Princeton University Press.
4. Jung, C. G. (1981). *Aion: Researches into the Phenomenology of the Self.* Princeton University Press.
    Jung, C. G. (1921). *Psychological Types.* Princeton University Press.
5. Peterson, J. B. (1999). *Maps of Meaning: The Architecture of Belief.* Routledge.
6. Peterson, J. B. (1999). *Maps of Meaning: The Architecture of Belief.* Routledge. Jung, C. G. (1981). *Aion: Researches into the Phenomenology of the Self.* Princeton University Press.
7. Peterson, J. B. (1999). *Maps of Meaning: The Architecture of Belief.* Routledge.
8. van der Kolk, B. (2014). *The Body Keeps the Score: Brain, Mind, and Body in the Healing of Trauma.* Viking.
9. van der Kolk, B. (2014). *The Body Keeps the Score: Brain, Mind, and Body in the Healing of Trauma.* Viking.
10. Litz, B. T., Stein, N., Delaney, E., Lebowitz, L., Nash, W. P., Silva, C., & Maguen, S. (2009). Moral injury and moral repair in war veterans: A preliminary model and intervention strategy. *Clinical Psychology Review,* 29(8), 695-706.
11. Litz, B. T., Stein, N., Delaney, E., Lebowitz, L., Nash, W. P., Silva, C., & Maguen, S. (2009). Moral injury and moral repair in war veterans: A preliminary model and intervention strategy. *Clinical Psychology Review,* 29(8), 695-706.
12. Litz, B. T., Stein, N., Delaney, E., Lebowitz, L., Nash, W. P., Silva, C., & Maguen, S. (2009). Moral injury and moral repair in war veterans: A preliminary model and intervention strategy. *Clinical Psychology Review,* 29(8), 695-706.
13. Litz, B. T., Stein, N., Delaney, E., Lebowitz, L., Nash, W. P., Silva, C., & Maguen, S. (2009). Moral injury and moral repair in war veterans: A preliminary model and intervention strategy. *Clinical Psychology Review,* 29(8), 695-706.

14. Litz, B. T., Stein, N., Delaney, E., Lebowitz, L., Nash, W. P., Silva, C., & Maguen, S. (2009). Moral injury and moral repair in war veterans: A preliminary model and intervention strategy. *Clinical Psychology Review*, 29(8), 695-706.
15. Litz, B. T., Stein, N., Delaney, E., Lebowitz, L., Nash, W. P., Silva, C., & Maguen, S. (2009). Moral injury and moral repair in war veterans: A preliminary model and intervention strategy. *Clinical Psychology Review*, 29(8), 695-706.

1. When it All Began

1. Felitti, V. J., Anda, R. F., Nordenberg, D., Williamson, D. F., Spitz, A. M., Edwards, V., Koss, M. P., & Marks, J. S. (1998). Relationship of childhood abuse and household dysfunction to many of the leading causes of death in adults: The Adverse Childhood Experiences (ACE) Study. American Journal of Preventive Medicine, 14(4), 245-258. doi:10.1016/S0749-3797(98)00017-8

Printed in the USA
CPSIA information can be obtained
at www.ICGtesting.com
CBHW031923221024
16238CB00011B/206